Yoga for Beginners:

60 Basic Yoga Poses for Flexibility, Stress Relief, and Inner Peace

D1166007

Susan Neal RN, MBA, MHS

Please consult with a healthcare professional before performing yoga postures or any new type of exercise program. If you have a special medical condition, you should consult with your doctor regarding possible modification of the program contained in this book. The author assumes no responsibility for any injury that may result from performing these yoga poses.

Copyright 2016, by Susan Neal

Published by Christian Yoga, LLC

ISBN-13: 978-0997763638

ISBN-10: 0997763639

Photography: RK Photos http://rkphotos1.zenfolio.com/

Cover Design: Angie Alaya

Yoga Posture Models: Susan Neal, Brooke Neal, Shelby Neal, and Callie Neal

I created a Beginner Yoga Class video for you, so you can watch how to perform many of the yoga poses in this book. Enjoy the free Beginner Yoga Class here: http://christianyoga.com/BeginnerYogaVideo

Table of Contents

Introduction

Thank you for downloading this book. I am Susan Neal, a certified yoga instructor with over 30 years of experience practicing and teaching yoga. I am a Registered Nurse with a Master of Health Science, and I love to teach people how to perform yoga and get healthy.

Popular culture depicts yoga as an exercise by individuals who get into pretzel-like positions that only one percent of the population can do. Have you ever bought a yoga DVD which was too advanced? Don't worry; this book will give you the satisfaction of knowing you can do yoga!

It does not have to be difficult. I will be teaching you a gentle set of yoga postures almost anyone can perform with practice. It may encourage you to know I have students in their 70s participating in my classes.

Detailed instructions on how to perform each position are illustrated with full-page photographs taken on the sugar-white sand dunes of the Emerald Coast of Florida. Sixty yoga postures provide a broad range of options from which to choose, from beginner to advanced. I have included warm-up stretches which gently relax the muscles and increase flexibility before performing the poses. Additionally, a series of three different yoga classes from beginner through intermediate levels provide variety to the routines. As your yoga practice advances, this book will continue to guide you into intermediate level positions.

After a brief overview of the origins and benefits of yoga, you will find a review of the essential components of yoga, a summary of what you will need to get started, and a section on injury prevention and posture modification if needed.

I am very excited that you have chosen to improve your health through performing yoga. I will share with you what I have learned about health and nutrition through my 30-year journey such as how to obtain your optimal weight through healthy eating. This is not about dieting. It is about lifestyle choices. Chapter 15 is about nutrition and contains a wealth of practical information and guidelines, such as tips on the causes of sugar and carbohydrate cravings and feasible solutions for controlling them. However, I am going to start this book with my story of how I lost my health and the steps I took to regain it. I hope you enjoy improving your overall health.

Chapter 1

WHEN I LOST MY HEALTH

In 2010, I was in excellent health at the age of 49. In November of that year, I had a crown placed on a tooth. Little did I know how that would mark the beginning of losing my good health. Ultimately, over the next nine months, this tooth abscessed and poisoned my body which resulted in ten different medical diagnoses.

One month after the crown, I began having two periods every month. This continued and eventually, 15 months later, I had surgery to remove two uterine polyps.

Two months later, I started experiencing depression, and I craved chocolate. In fact, where I used to eat one or two candy bars per year, I now ate one square of Ghirardelli chocolate every evening.

In March 2011, I was diagnosed with an ovarian cyst and, two months later, adrenal fatigue. Although exhausted all the time, I had difficulty sleeping. By now, I should have known that something was wrong with my body. However, I didn't realize it even though, as a yoga instructor, I teach my clients to be more in tune with their body.

My doctor who diagnosed the adrenal fatigue prescribed three different adrenal vitamins five times a day. That's 15 vitamin pills per day! The physician also prescribed progesterone cream for a hormonal imbalance as I was in peri-menopause. That summer I could not even attend my aunt's funeral because I did not have the energy to fly across the country for a long trip.

In July, I had flashes of light in my left eye when I quickly turned my head to the left. This was from a hole in my retina that was diagnosed and treated with laser surgery two months later.

In August, I began experiencing visual migraines even though I had never suffered from headaches. That month, I went to my dentist for a cleaning and I told them I had a bump above one of my teeth. They said that is never a good sign. The tooth that I had crowned back in November had abscessed and was draining all of the putrid fluid into my gastrointestinal system. I had an emergency root canal along with ten days of antibiotics and two weeks of steroids. Afterward, I was so exhausted I could not even put away the groceries after shopping. No one understood how depleted my system was because on the outside I looked fine. However, on the inside, I was a train wreck.

In September, I had laser surgery on my eye. My doctor also found I was anemic, and my vitamin D level was low.

In the fall, I continued to be very sick. Since my doctors were unable to do much for me, I tried alternative healthcare therapies such as massage, acupuncture, and colonic therapy. My colonic therapist found a Candida infection in my colon. I had never heard of this type of infection before, so my therapist gave me *The Body Ecology Diet* by Donna Gates. The information in this book confirmed that I had an overgrowth of Candida in my gastrointestinal system. I followed the steps outlined in this book to get rid of the infection.

I turned 50 that August, and I had lost my health. For 50 years, I had taken for granted my good health. Now I realized it was precious. Ultimately, what had occurred in my body was a poisoning from my abscessed tooth resulting in ten different medical diagnoses in the following order:

1. Bi-monthly periods caused by uterine polyps

2. Depression

3. Ovarian cyst

4. Adrenal fatigue *?? me: tooth problem?*

5. Hormonal imbalance

6. Retinal tear

7. Visual migraine

8. Anemia

9. Low vitamin D level

10. Candidiasis infection of my colon

For the following eight months, I struggled to regain my health. To eradicate the Candida, I stopped eating most fruits, rice, flour, sugar, and desserts. I lost ten pounds. During this time, I would take one step forward and two steps back, then three steps forward and one step back. It was a slow process, but, after eight months of being on the strict diet, I finally regained my health. While I was sick, I continued to teach several yoga classes a week. My yoga practice aided my healing process.

In July 2012, I felt like I was healed. The Body Ecology Diet that I was on for eight months required great self-control, but I was determined to succeed because I desperately wanted my health back. Ultimately, I beat the Candida infection in my gut and restored my adrenal glands. We have glorious bodies that will heal themselves if we give them the right building blocks.

Chapter 2

ORIGINS OF YOGA

The earliest evidence of yoga dates back to around 3000 BCE in stone impressions of figures depicting yoga postures found in the Indus Valley Civilization (currently Pakistan and northwest India). These stone seals were excavated by a team led by John Marshall in 1928-29.

The term "yoga" was introduced around 1500 BCE when the Hindus began incorporating it into their religion. Buddhism began its association with yoga through the use of physical postures and meditation around 600 BCE. However, the archeological evidence from the stone seals suggests yoga predates the world's three great religions: Hinduism, Buddhism, and Christianity.

The most popular type of yoga in the United States is Hatha Yoga, which does not include the Eastern religion or the philosophical portion of yoga. Instead, it focuses on the physical aspects of the body which, in turn, influences us psychologically. This book focuses on Hatha Yoga.

Without even realizing it, we store stress within our bodies. Feel the tight muscles on your shoulders. Usually, we ignore this tension, but it builds up within us. Holding yoga poses releases this tension, clearing our minds and making us feel better! The movements recharge us, making us feel more alert, yet peaceful. At the same time, we are building strength and endurance. A strong body positively influences the mind. You feel better about yourself physically and, therefore, psychologically.

Hatha Yoga strengthens the mind through focused breathing and meditation, so the body and mind work in harmony. The yoga movements lead to a calm, focused mind and a strong, flexible body that makes one feel peaceful.

Chapter 3

STRESS RELIEF

It is hard to keep up with today's fast-paced world and changing technology. From the time you wake up in the morning until you go to bed at night, you are pulled in many different directions and exposed to all sorts of non-ionizing radiation from electronic devices. This causes stress, which is a factor in all of our lives. How does stress affect you physically? You may experience tense, aching muscles; find yourself becoming tired and irritable; develop high blood pressure; or become anxious and worried. Many people, subsequently, exercise less and eat poorly. It is time to start taking care of yourself!

When performing yoga, you focus on breathing and quiet the mind, allowing worries to drift away. As the muscles stretch, tension is released which improves flexibility and decreases joint and muscle stiffness. This gentle stretching also calms the spirit.

The practice of yoga integrates the three aspects of self: body, mind, and spirit. Yoga has been found to ease the symptoms of many chronic conditions such as asthma, arthritis, chronic fatigue syndrome, high blood pressure, and chronic back pain.

My years as a healthcare administrator at Mayo Clinic Jacksonville managing over 140 staff members were very stressful. Exhausted in the evenings, I would come home and lay on the couch while my husband cooked dinner. Fortunately and providentially, two nights a week we attended a yoga class which renewed my body and mind. Afterward, I felt energized and could even cook dinner! I was amazed by the stress reduction provided by yoga. You too can experience the same results.

Chapter 4

HEALTH BENEFITS OF YOGA

Many people today have a disconnection within their body, preventing it from working to its full potential. Stress, brain fog, muscle pain, and poor metabolism are just a few symptoms that result from this disconnection. Are you being held back from your full potential? Chronic disease and being overweight are typical for many people today, but that does not have to be the norm. Yoga will help your body function better, and you will become healthier!

Look at the benefits of performing yoga:

Enhances Muscles Tone, Definition, Strength, and Physical Fitness

Muscles become well-defined, and the additional strength helps to prevent injuries.

Increases Range of Motion in Joints

Seniors in my yoga class say that yoga prevents muscle and joint stiffness, and they rarely miss a class.

Prevents Cartilage and Joint Breakdown

The full range of motion performed during the poses supports joints.

Enhances Coordination and Improves Reaction Time

Muscles become stronger and leaner, and your balance, coordination, and even reaction time improve.

Increases Overall Flexibility

The flexibility of your spine improves your posture, which makes you look younger! It also keeps the spinal discs supple.

Relieves Muscle Pain and Tension

Stretching muscles, ligaments, and tendons reduces muscle pain and tension.

Eases Pain

Several medical studies have shown that yoga reduces back pain, arthritis, fibromyalgia, and other chronic conditions. One of my clients told me that she took less pain medicine for fibromyalgia the days she attended a yoga class.

Eases Stress, Tension, and Anxiety

Yoga creates inner peace, so perform yoga instead of taking anti-anxiety medication.

Improves Depression

Some studies have found yoga increases serotonin levels, which makes you feel happier!

Improves Memory

Focusing on the breath and the present moment, through meditation, enhances concentration, and memory.

Eases Migraines

Yoga has been found to help with migraines, so try yoga before medication.

Deepens Sleep

No more tossing and turning, just sound sleep.

Improves Lung Function

Usually one does not think about respiration, but during yoga class you do. In turn, this enhancement gives you more energy and vitality!

Improves Circulation

Exercise increases the heart rate, and this delivers more oxygen to the whole body.

Lowers Blood Pressure

Medical studies have proven that doing yoga decreases blood pressure.

Reduces Blood Sugar

Studies have shown diabetics' blood sugar drop through the practice of yoga.

Reduces Bad Cholesterol (LDL) and Boosts Good Cholesterol (HDL)

Studies have demonstrated that the practice of yoga can decrease LDL and increase HDL.

Improves Metabolism

Have you ever thought your metabolism does not work as well as it should? Give it a jump start with yoga.

Relaxes the Body Systems

Focusing on deep breathing throughout the session increases blood flow to all internal organs which lowers breathing and heart rate.

Boosts Immunity

Many of the yoga postures stimulate the lymph system to drain toxins out of the body, which heightens immunity.

When you feel better about yourself, you will make healthier choices and begin reaching your ideal weight. In fact, most people think I am ten years younger than my actual age. I attribute that to practicing yoga for over 30 years. So look younger, feel better, and do yoga!

This is me in my mid-50s.

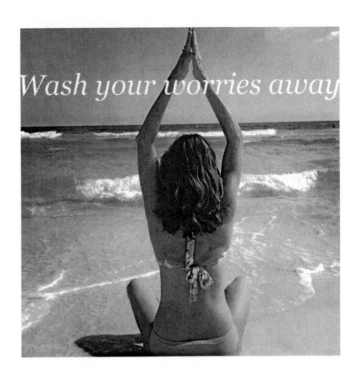

Chapter 5

ESSENTIAL COMPONENTS OF YOGA: BREATHING, STRETCHING, AND MEDITATION

Three essential components of yoga are breathing, stretching in the yoga posture, and meditating.

Breathing

Breathing is an essential element of yoga. We do not usually think about breathing, much less concentrate on breathing deeply. However, moving additional oxygen into your cells will make you feel better and give you more energy. Always focus on your breathing during all of the yoga postures. Your entire body will benefit. Imagine your lungs are a balloon and this balloon expands and deflates entirely with each inhalation and exhalation.

Recently, I went to the doctor and had a pulse oximeter placed on my index finger. The oxygen level in my blood was 94%. I thought it was low even though the medical assistant said 94-100% was normal. The following week, at my chiropractor, I took several deep breaths before they placed the pulse oximeter on my finger. This time, my oxygen level was 100%. I brought up the oxygen level of my blood 6% just by breathing deeply!

An excellent way to ascertain how long to hold a yoga posture is by counting the number of breaths. A breath is a complete cycle of inhaling and exhaling. One should stay in most positions for three to five breaths. Each yoga pose description in Chapters 7 through 12 contains the optimal number of breaths desired while holding the pose.

Stretching

Flexibility is the ability to move our muscles and joints through a complete range of motion. Stretching stimulates the production of tissue lubricants which help the muscles rebuild with healthy tissue. Additional benefits of stretching include joint lubrication, improved healing, better circulation, and enhanced mobility.

When you stretch to the edge of discomfort, it can elicit feelings of pain. Therefore, you should slowly allow your muscles to release their tightness, then gently push further into the posture at your own pace. When you stay in a stretch for at least 20 seconds, you enable your connective tissues to become more elastic.

Stretching and breathing are interrelated in the yoga movements. As you inhale, your muscles tighten slightly, but, as you exhale, they seem to grow longer and you are able to push further into the pose. The exhalation relaxes the muscles which facilitates the stretch. Once engaged in the full posture, you may experience a pleasant moment of inner peace. Relaxation follows and your stretching is enhanced, as well as your sense of well-being. Now that you are breathing deeply and stretching all the muscles in your body, you will discover your stress dissipates, allowing you to recapture inner harmony.

Meditation

Rarely do we allow ourselves meditative time to be quiet and think, or spend time with our Creator. As we do so, meditation also enhances our brain function. Numerous scientific studies have revealed increased brain activity occurs during meditation. Meditation decreases perceived stress: improves psychological well-being, memory, and cognitive performance. As an article from the *Huffington Post* states, "A UCLA team of neuroscientists found that a three-month course of yoga and meditation helped minimize the cognitive and emotional problems that often precede Alzheimer's disease and other forms of dementia." As you can tell, meditation is a superb form of exercise for the brain.

We go to the gym to exercise our physical bodies and we perform aerobic training to work our heart. So why don't we perform exercises for the brain? Meditation enhances brain function, and this is very important with the rise in the occurrence of dementia and Alzheimer's.

Yoga prepares the mind for the meditative session by releasing tension from our bodies and minds, allowing us to go deeper into meditation. This involves training your mind through acknowledging its content without becoming wrapped up in what you are thinking. Through focusing the mind, your concentration increases. Some of the benefits of meditation for well-being include increasing happiness and contentment while decreasing anxiety, worry, and fear. Meditation benefits the physical body through lowering blood pressure and improving memory.

I will explain each of the following methods of meditation: breathing practices, guided relaxation, guided imagery, affirmations, and stillness.

Breathing Practices

Focusing on your breath while performing yoga movements is essential. The deep inhalation and complete exhalation oxygenates and detoxifies the body, making you feel better and giving you more energy. Imagine your lungs are a balloon. Blow up the balloon to its maximum capacity and thoroughly deflate it. This will calm your nerves and clarify your mind. While in the relaxation portion of the yoga class, choose to focus on your breath. Notice how your chest rises and falls with each inhalation and exhalation or you can focus on the breath moving in and out of your nostrils. This calms your mind.

Guided Relaxation

This is performed through relaxing your entire body from your head to your toes by paying attention to various parts of your body in slow movements down your torso. The relaxation session releases tension and relaxes the body, mind, emotions, and spirit. I have included a guided relaxation segment at the end of Chapter 14. Another form of guided relaxation includes tensing and then relaxing each part of your body beginning with your head and moving down your torso. For example, tense your facial muscles for three seconds then slowly release this tension and feel the muscles relax completely. Move to the next area of your body such as your neck and so on.

Guided Imagery

Guided imagery is performed after the guided relaxation session at the end of the class. Choose to focus on something such as a leaf floating down a slow-moving stream. Follow this leaf as it continues to move on top of the water. If you become distracted, bring your focus back to the floating leaf. A second example includes focusing on an area of your body that needs repair, such as a hamstring injury. Visualize the torn hamstring and imagine cells within your body repairing the tendon. This may enhance healing of that area of your body. Thirdly, you could focus on ocean waves. In your mind, follow a wave as it flows onto the shore, then focus on the next wave. To enhance this experience, listen to music with the sounds of the ocean. If you are listening to instrumental music, you could imagine the hands that are playing the instrument, such as fingers gliding over the keyboard of a piano.

Affirmations

The meditative technique of using affirmations includes repeating or pondering brief uplifting statements. Personally, I focus on Scripture. This can be performed while holding a yoga position or during the relaxation/meditative session at the end of the class. These positive proclamations counteract negative thoughts and feelings while increasing inner strength and energy.

Stillness

Stillness involves focusing the mind on nothing, like a blank slate. I find this to be the most difficult type of meditation to perform. Center your mind on stillness, silence, and peace. Your mind will wander but each time deliberately bring your thoughts back to stillness at that present moment. Realize that it is normal for your mind to wander, so do not get upset with yourself. Instead, understand that this is training your mind. Just like beginning any physical activity, you should begin slowly with three-to-five minute sessions and build up to 20 minutes. With time, your mind will wander less and less. The meditative technique of stillness nurtures the spirit while calming the mind and emotions. It also provides mental clarity and perspective. Meditation is the practice of contemplation. It is the focusing of the mind, especially on God. Many times, meditation will lead to insights, solutions to problems, and profound spiritual wisdom.

How to Begin

To begin your yoga practice, you will need loose-fitting clothes and a yoga mat or towel. It is that simple; it does not have to be difficult. I have new clients in their 60s who learn how to do yoga with ease, and you can too!

Make sure to drink plenty of water (only) after performing yoga, but not during the yoga session. Don't eat a heavy meal before doing yoga either. In fact, it is best to have an empty stomach.

Now that we have reviewed the key elements of yoga and what you need, let's get started.

Chapter 6

INJURY PREVENTION AND POSE MODIFICATION

How to Avoid Injuries:

- Do not wear socks; you could slip.

- Make sure there is enough space to move freely into the poses without hitting something.

- Always perform the 15-20 minutes of warm-up stretches that are included before the yoga poses. Warm-ups stretch all the muscles in the body and prepare one for the yoga postures.

- Do not force yourself further into a stretch than what your body would naturally do. It is better to allow time (20 seconds or more) and gravity to bring you further into the pose than to push yourself prematurely.

- Don't compare yourself to anyone else. Yoga is not a competition. After performing yoga for 30 years, I still have to stretch thoroughly before I can touch my toes. We all have an edge of tension, and you should stop at your edge. It does not matter if someone else can put their hand flat on the floor and you can barely touch the floor with your fingertips.

- Be careful of your wrists. If you have weak wrists, modify or do not perform these poses: Plank, Downward Dog, and Cobra. I have an old wrist injury from gardening, so I am cautious about doing poses where I must hold up my body weight.

- Do not do yoga when you have a severe musculoskeletal injury. Allow your injury to heal. If you give yourself time, the injured area of you body will heal much faster than if you push yourself to do too much too quickly.

- Modify yoga postures if you are having difficulty performing the pose. Modification suggestions are listed at the end of this chapter.

- Attend a yoga class and ask for help from the instructor.

- Buy a yoga DVD (Here is a link to two DVDs I produced: http://christianyoga.com/).

Yoga Pose Modification

When performing yoga postures, keep the movements slow and focused. Allow gravity to bring you further into the pose. Do not force yourself. Never go past the point of slight tension when in a pose. Listen to your body: if it tells you to come out of a posture early, do so. Become attuned to what your body is saying and don't ignore it.

Yoga positions can easily be modified. As an example, for a cross-legged position, simply extend the legs in front of you while bending your knees instead of crossing them if you have problems with your knees. If you have lower back problems, modify the Cobra by keeping the forearms instead of the hands on the ground, so your back is not stretched as far. Feel free to adjust a posture to meet your physical limitations. Remember to listen to your body: don't force it and modify as needed.

Here is a list of yoga posture modifications. In addition, I have placed modifications at the beginning of each chapter that contains those poses.

Yoga Posture Modification Suggestions

Cross-legged pose—extend the legs in front of you while bending your knees instead of crossing your legs.

Downward Dog—move into the Half-Dog where you stay on your knees and forearms while lifting your tailbone up.

Camel—from a kneeling position, sit on your heels and place your palms flat on the floor behind you with fingertips pointed away from your body. Lift your pelvis so you have a straight line between your knees, neck, and head.

Dancer—stand in front of a wall so your fingertips touch the wall as you lean forward into the pose.

Cobra—keep your forearms on the mat while lifting your upper torso. This modified Cobra is called the Sphinx pose.

Plank—keep your forearms on the mat when moving into the Plank. This decreases the pressure on your wrists.

Bridge—stay in the basic pose of the Bridge; therefore, do not clasp your hands together under your back.

Shoulder Stand—only lift your legs up into the air, not your pelvis. Then perform the ankle movements.

Fish—do not tilt your head back; instead stay in the basic posture of the Fish with your upper torso weight on your elbows.

Chapter 7

60 BASIC YOGA POSTURES

I teach a gentle, beginner-intermediate yoga class. Listed below are three different yoga sessions incorporating 60 yoga poses. Be sure to perform the warm-up stretches as indicated in the outline below before beginning the more challenging yoga postures, to prepare your body for the more difficult movements. As with any fitness routine, be sure to check with a doctor before performing these yoga postures. Also, a posture index is included at the back of this book for reference.

I created a Beginner Yoga Class video for you which includes the postures listed in the Gentle Yoga Posture Session below. You can access that video here:(http://christianyoga.com/BeginnerYogaVideo)

Gentle Yoga Posture Session

Cross Legged	Bent Knee Seated Forward Fold
Chin to Chest	Seated Forward Bend
Ear to Shoulder	Seated Spinal Twist
Head Turns	Lion
Sun Breath	Table
Upper Body Stretching	Cat and Dog Stretch
Elbow to Knee	Thread the Needle
Seated Open-Angle Pose/Forward Bend	Pigeon
	Yoga Mudra
Seated Open-Angle Side Bend	Cleansing Breath
Revolved Head-to-Knee Pose	Squat
Butterfly	Standing Forward Bend

Mountain
Half-Moon Side Bend
Standing Abdominal Lifts
Warrior I
Triangle
Tree
Half-Locust
Cobra
Locust
Bow
Child's Pose

Double Leg Raises
Supine Reach Through (Variation)
Bridge
Shoulder Stand
Fish
Lying Spinal Twist (One Leg Variation)
Alternate Nostril Breath
Corpse Pose
Knee Hug

Intermediate I Yoga Posture Session (same as gentle series except)

Add Shoulder Shrug/Circles
Add Staff Pose
Add Camel
Add Kegel
Standing Side Yoga Mudra instead of kneeling Yoga Mudra
Warrior II instead of Triangle
Warrior III instead of Tree
Boat instead of Double Leg Raises
Single Knee Hug instead of Knee Hug

Intermediate II Yoga Posture Session (same as gentle series except)

Cow Face instead of Thread the Needle
Add Low Lunge
Add Downward Dog
Add Plank
Add Standing Forward Bend with Leg Clasp and Halfway Lift
Posture Clasp instead of sitting Yoga Mudra
Dancer instead of Tree
Reclining Spinal Twist (Two Knee Variation) instead of Lying Spinal Twist

Chapter 8

UPPER-BODY STRETCHES

Be sure to perform the warm-up stretches listed in this chapter before undertaking the more difficult yoga postures. The stretches will loosen all the muscles in the body, which will decrease the possibility of injury. Remember to modify poses as needed.

Yoga Posture Modification Suggestions

Cross-legged pose-extend the legs in front of you while bending your knees instead of crossing your legs.

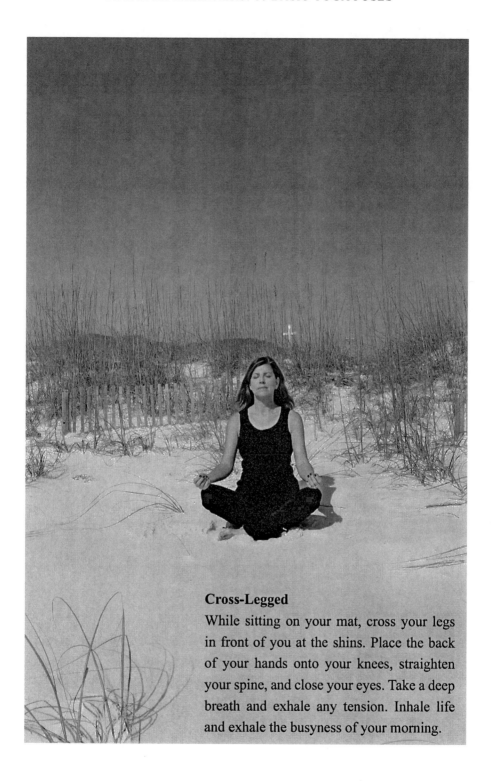

Cross-Legged

While sitting on your mat, cross your legs in front of you at the shins. Place the back of your hands onto your knees, straighten your spine, and close your eyes. Take a deep breath and exhale any tension. Inhale life and exhale the busyness of your morning.

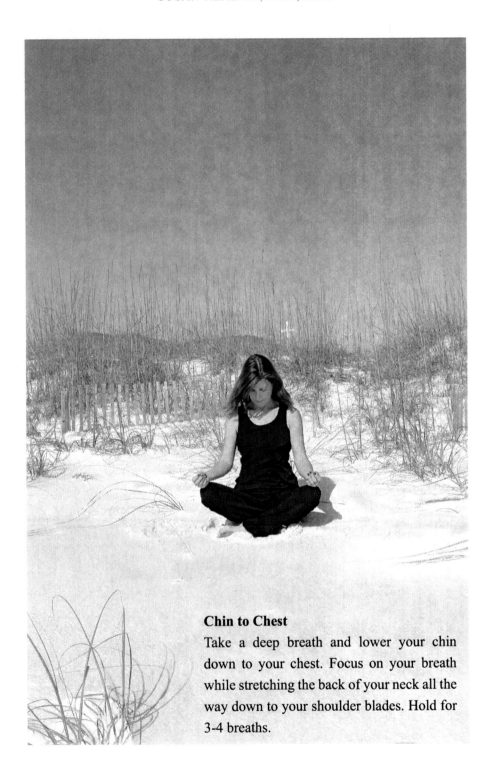

Chin to Chest

Take a deep breath and lower your chin down to your chest. Focus on your breath while stretching the back of your neck all the way down to your shoulder blades. Hold for 3-4 breaths.

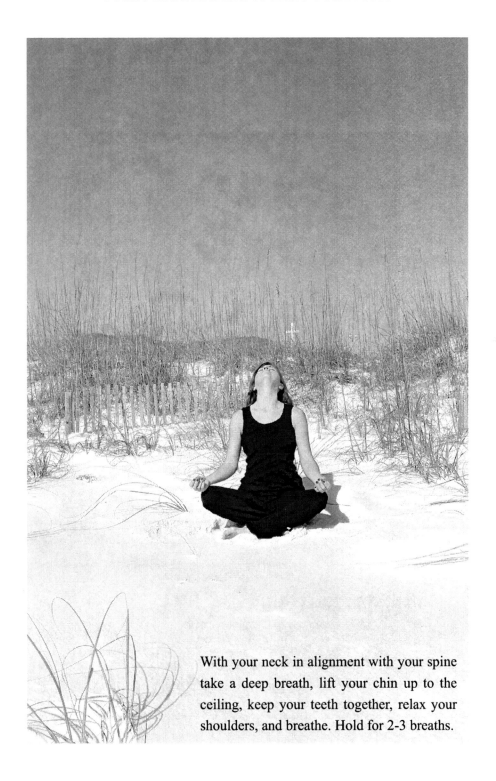

With your neck in alignment with your spine take a deep breath, lift your chin up to the ceiling, keep your teeth together, relax your shoulders, and breathe. Hold for 2-3 breaths.

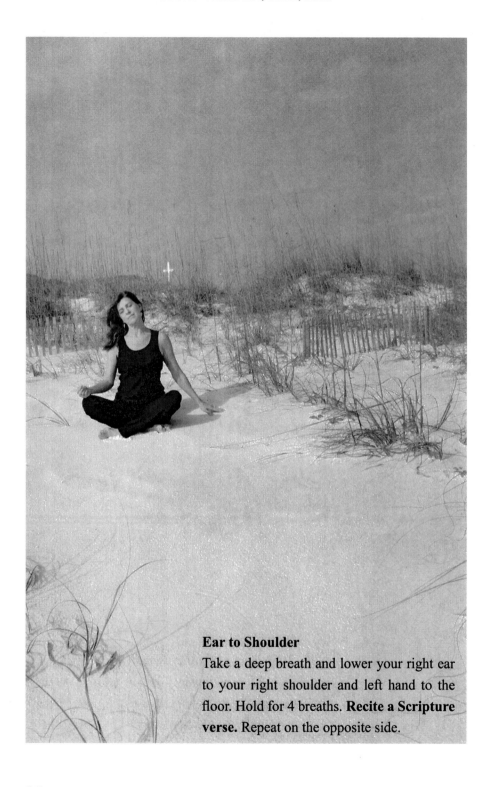

Ear to Shoulder
Take a deep breath and lower your right ear to your right shoulder and left hand to the floor. Hold for 4 breaths. **Recite a Scripture verse.** Repeat on the opposite side.

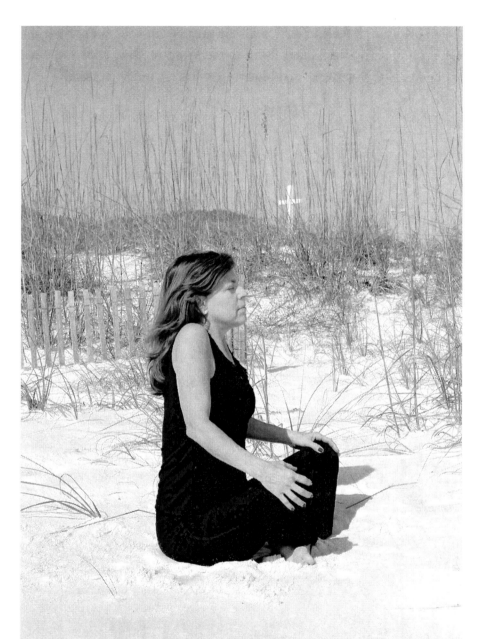

Shoulder Shrug and Circles

Inhale and lift your shoulders up toward your ears. Exhale and lower the shoulders. Repeat several times. Inhale and raise your shoulders toward your ears and rotate them forward in large circles and backward in circles.

Feel how good it feels to stretch all the muscles in your neck. Now is a time to quiet your mind and listen to the Word of God, allowing these words to enter your heart and bloom like flowers in Springtime.

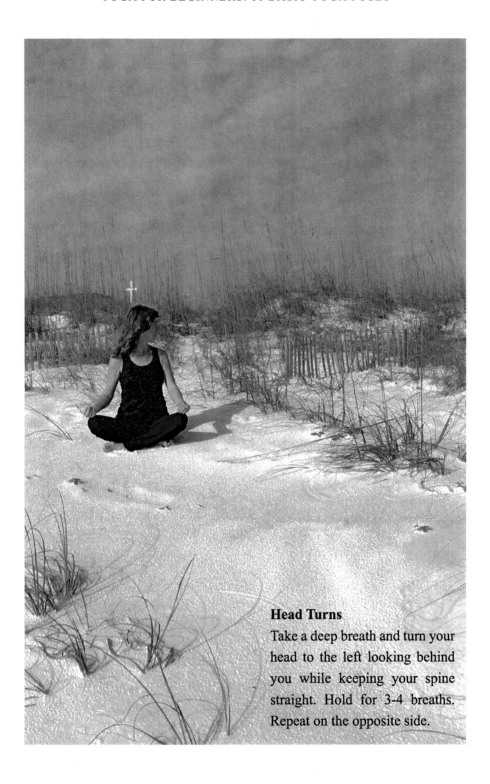

Head Turns
Take a deep breath and turn your head to the left looking behind you while keeping your spine straight. Hold for 3-4 breaths. Repeat on the opposite side.

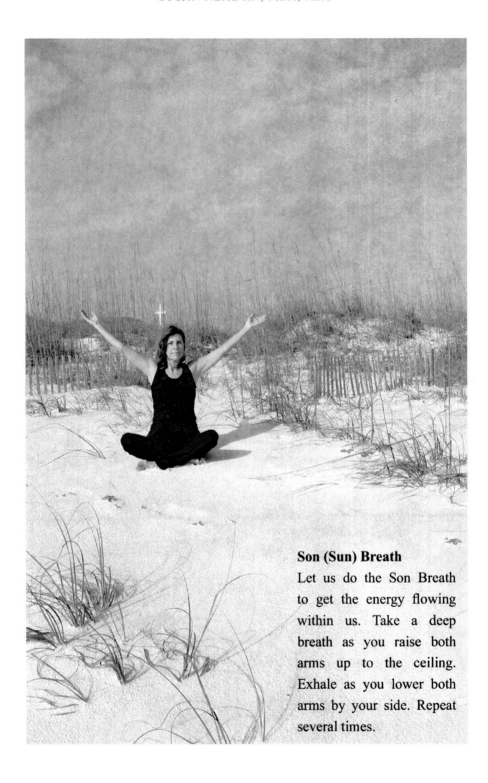

Son (Sun) Breath

Let us do the Son Breath to get the energy flowing within us. Take a deep breath as you raise both arms up to the ceiling. Exhale as you lower both arms by your side. Repeat several times.

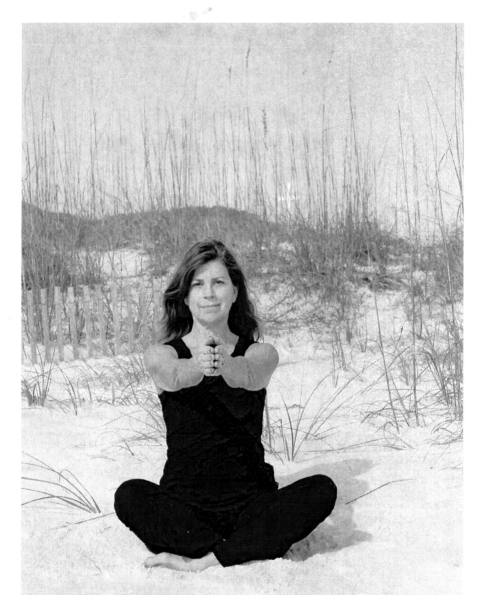

Upper Body Stretching

Now we will stretch our upper body. On an inhale, put your hands together in prayer position in front of your chest. Exhale, move your arms out in front of you, elbows straight, hands in a prayer position. Straighten your spine and neck, stretch through your shoulders, elbows, hands, and fingertips. **Recite a Scripture verse.**

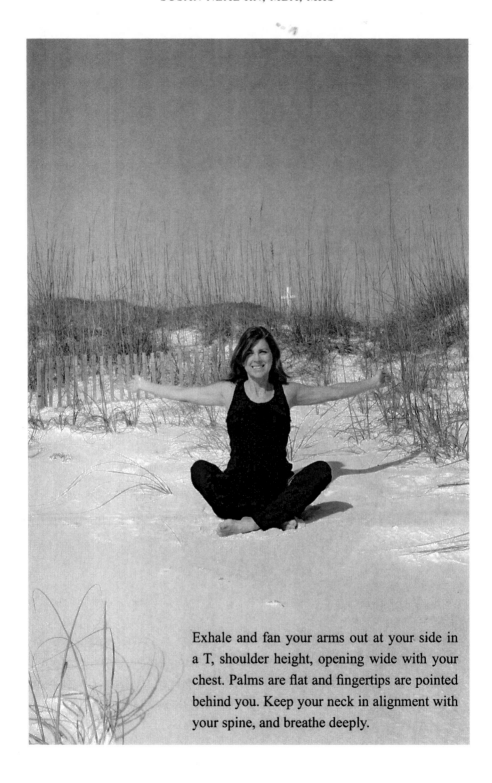

Exhale and fan your arms out at your side in a T, shoulder height, opening wide with your chest. Palms are flat and fingertips are pointed behind you. Keep your neck in alignment with your spine, and breathe deeply.

Remember to inhale and exhale deeply during all of the yoga postures. Many times we take a shallow breath. During this yoga class, focus on expanding your lungs fully like a balloon and exhaling completely.

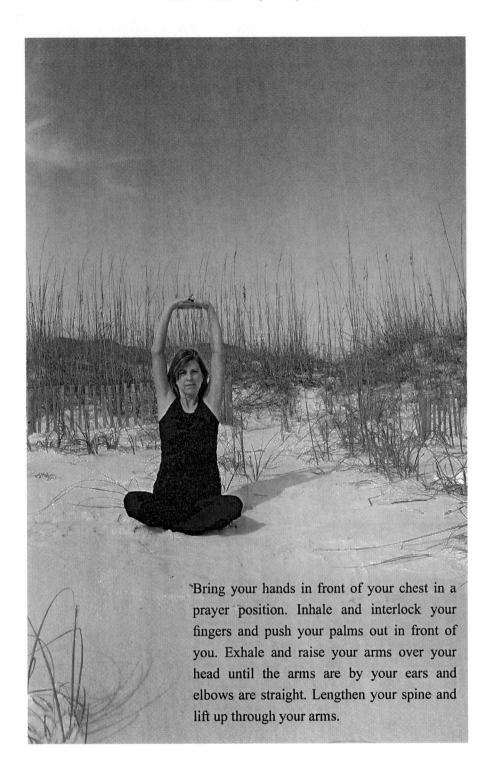

Bring your hands in front of your chest in a prayer position. Inhale and interlock your fingers and push your palms out in front of you. Exhale and raise your arms over your head until the arms are by your ears and elbows are straight. Lengthen your spine and lift up through your arms.

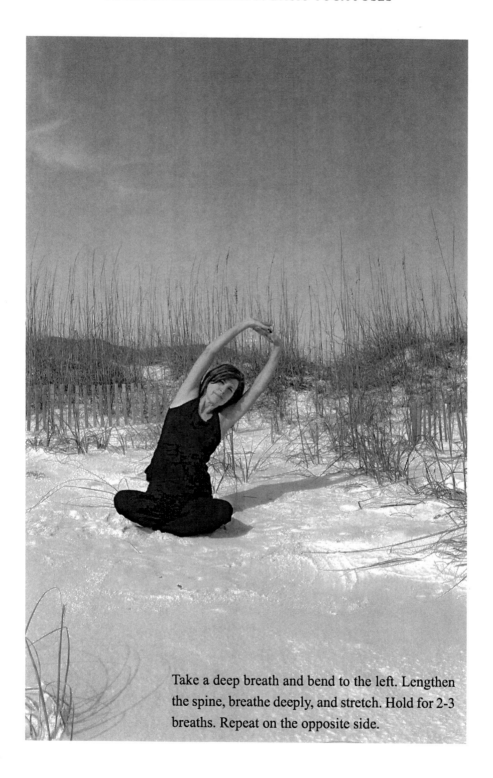

Take a deep breath and bend to the left. Lengthen the spine, breathe deeply, and stretch. Hold for 2-3 breaths. Repeat on the opposite side.

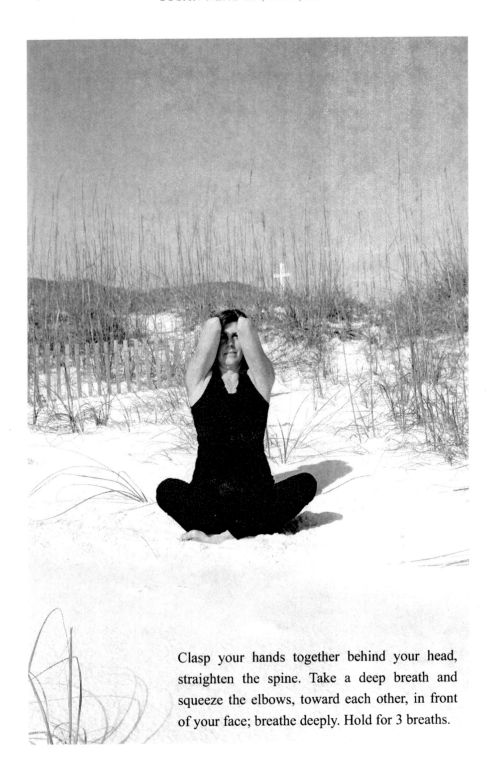

Clasp your hands together behind your head, straighten the spine. Take a deep breath and squeeze the elbows, toward each other, in front of your face; breathe deeply. Hold for 3 breaths.

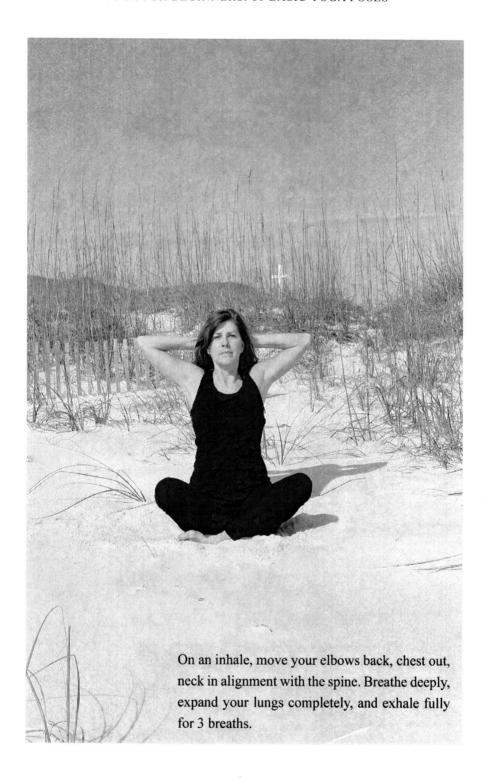

On an inhale, move your elbows back, chest out, neck in alignment with the spine. Breathe deeply, expand your lungs completely, and exhale fully for 3 breaths.

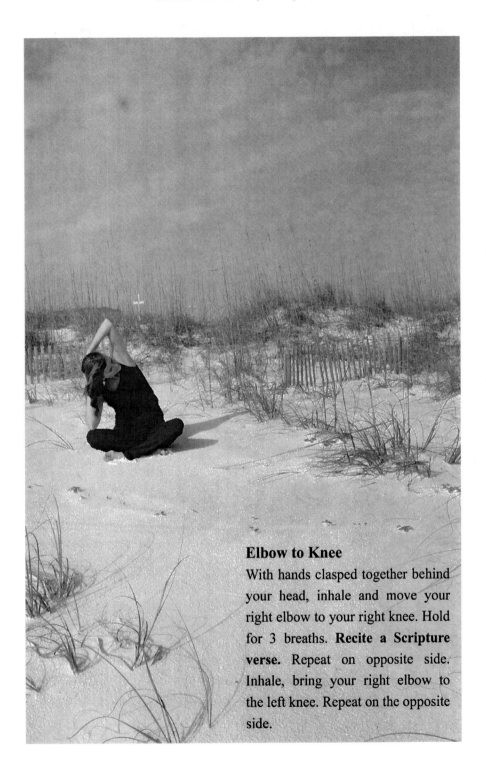

Elbow to Knee

With hands clasped together behind your head, inhale and move your right elbow to your right knee. Hold for 3 breaths. **Recite a Scripture verse.** Repeat on opposite side. Inhale, bring your right elbow to the left knee. Repeat on the opposite side.

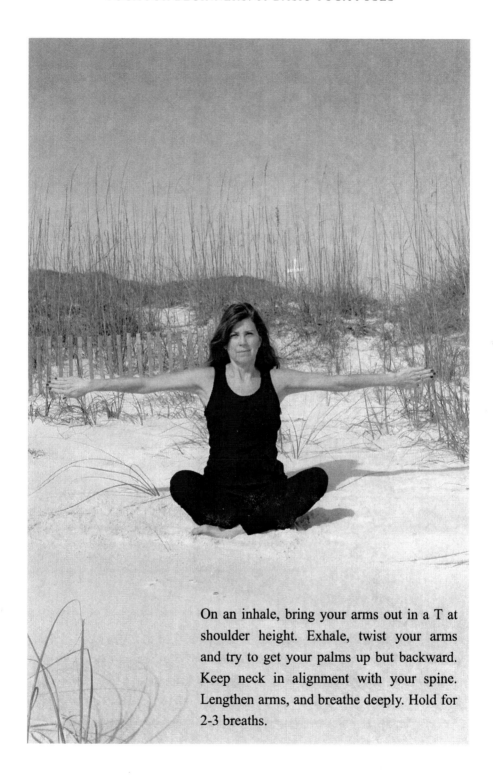

On an inhale, bring your arms out in a T at shoulder height. Exhale, twist your arms and try to get your palms up but backward. Keep neck in alignment with your spine. Lengthen arms, and breathe deeply. Hold for 2-3 breaths.

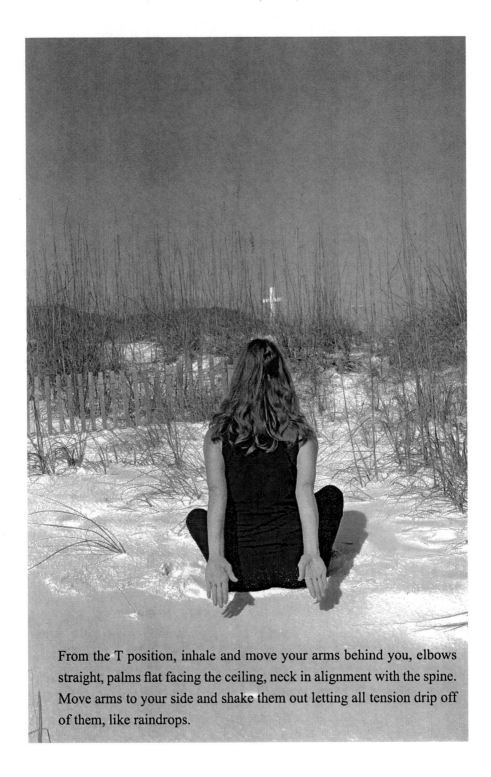

From the T position, inhale and move your arms behind you, elbows straight, palms flat facing the ceiling, neck in alignment with the spine. Move arms to your side and shake them out letting all tension drip off of them, like raindrops.

Cross-Legged

While sitting on your mat, cross your legs in front of you at the shins. Place your hands onto your knees, close your eyes and feel how good it feels to stretch the muscles in your neck, shoulders, arms, all the way down to your hands and fingertips. Now we will stretch our lower body as we have our upper body.

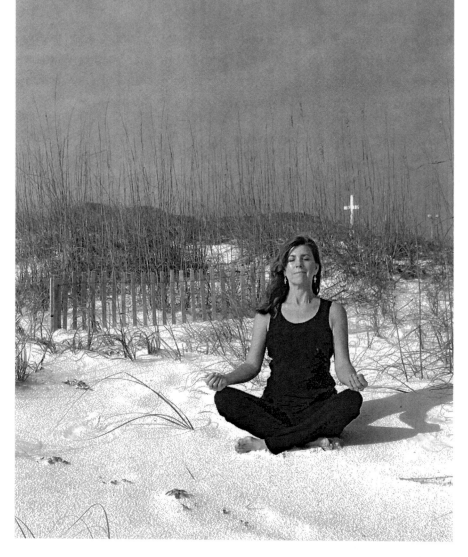

Chapter 9

LOWER-BODY STRETCHES

Now we will stretch our lower body as we have our upper body because it is important to stretch your entire body, from your head to your toes, before you begin the more challenging yoga postures. These stretches make you feel as though you have received a gentle massage.

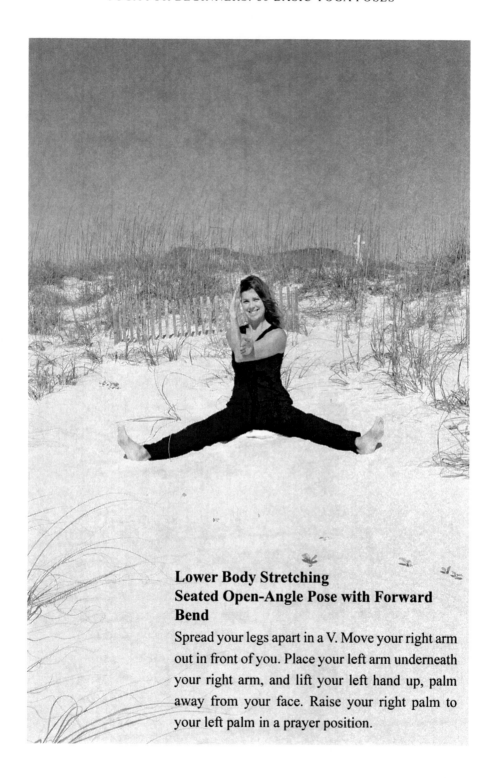

Lower Body Stretching
Seated Open-Angle Pose with Forward
Bend

Spread your legs apart in a V. Move your right arm out in front of you. Place your left arm underneath your right arm, and lift your left hand up, palm away from your face. Raise your right palm to your left palm in a prayer position.

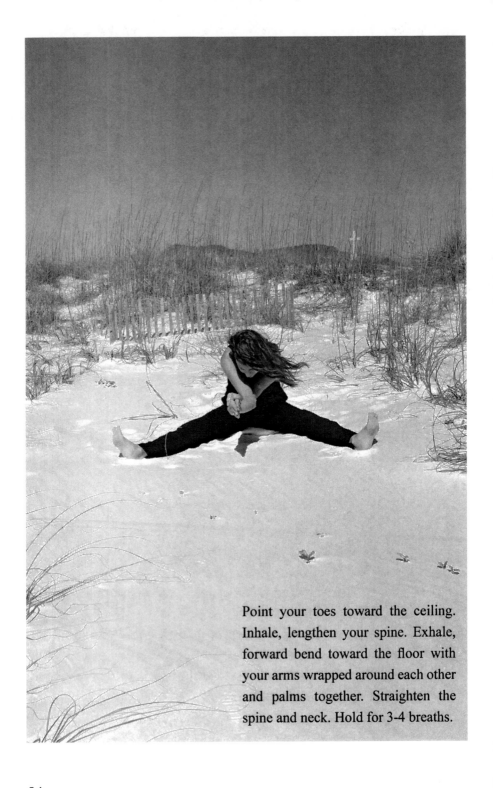

Point your toes toward the ceiling. Inhale, lengthen your spine. Exhale, forward bend toward the floor with your arms wrapped around each other and palms together. Straighten the spine and neck. Hold for 3-4 breaths.

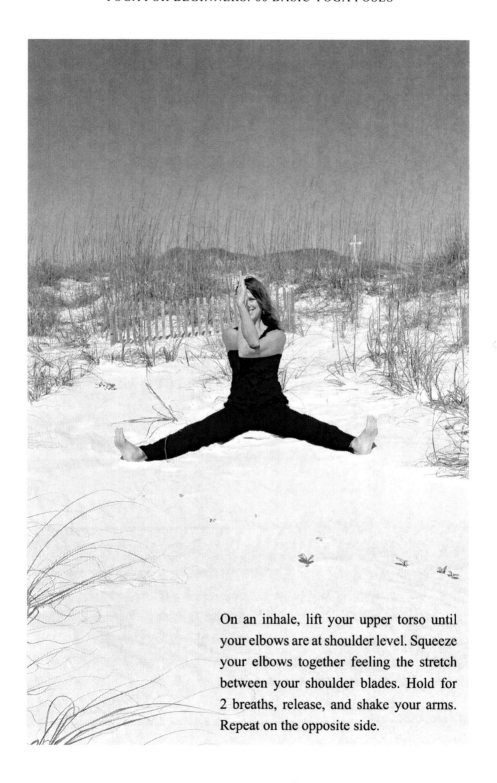

On an inhale, lift your upper torso until your elbows are at shoulder level. Squeeze your elbows together feeling the stretch between your shoulder blades. Hold for 2 breaths, release, and shake your arms. Repeat on the opposite side.

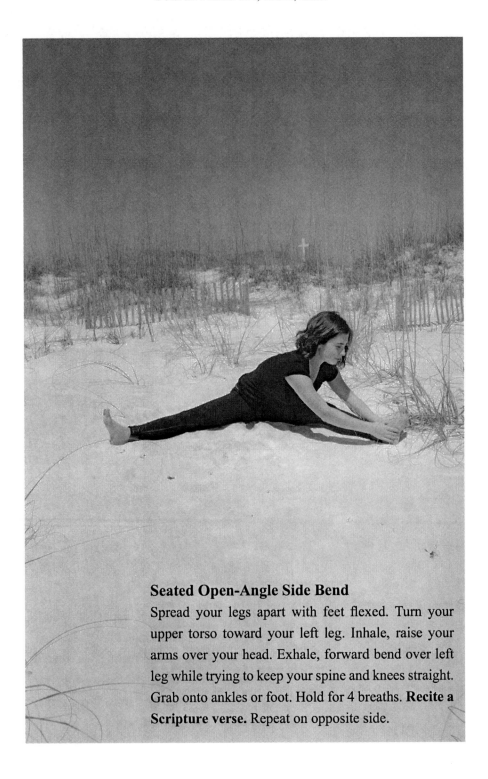

Seated Open-Angle Side Bend

Spread your legs apart with feet flexed. Turn your upper torso toward your left leg. Inhale, raise your arms over your head. Exhale, forward bend over left leg while trying to keep your spine and knees straight. Grab onto ankles or foot. Hold for 4 breaths. **Recite a Scripture verse.** Repeat on opposite side.

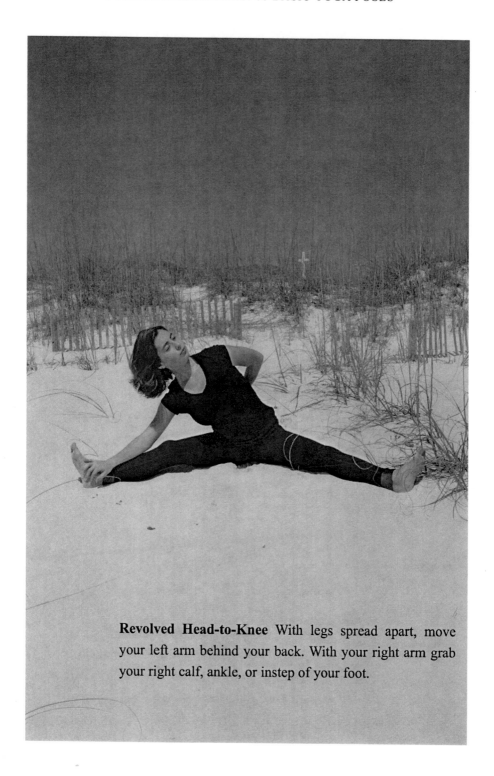

Revolved Head-to-Knee With legs spread apart, move your left arm behind your back. With your right arm grab your right calf, ankle, or instep of your foot.

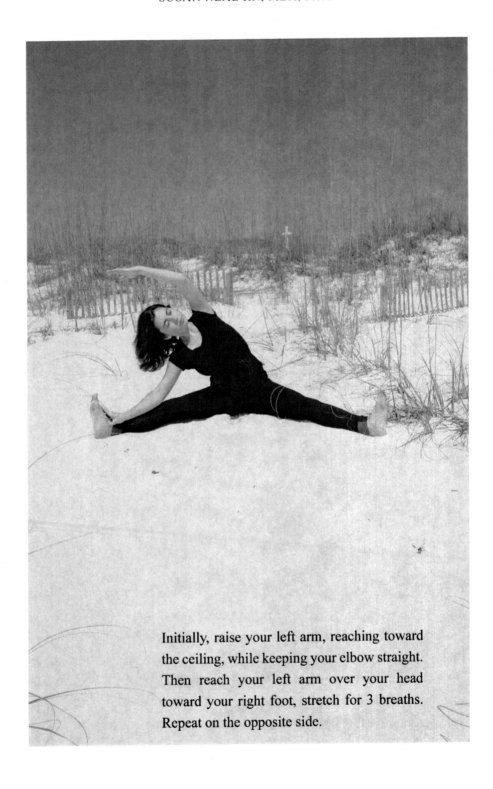

Initially, raise your left arm, reaching toward the ceiling, while keeping your elbow straight. Then reach your left arm over your head toward your right foot, stretch for 3 breaths. Repeat on the opposite side.

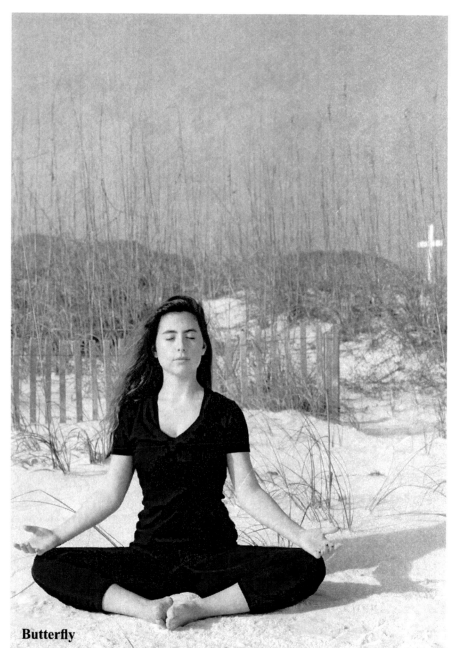

Butterfly
Put your feet together and flutter your knees. Inhale, lengthen your spine and neck; exhale, lower your knees down toward the floor and hold for 3 breaths.

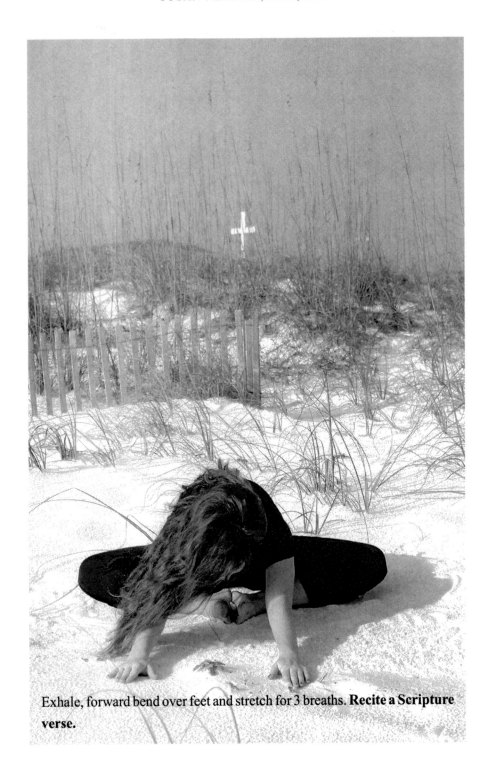

Exhale, forward bend over feet and stretch for 3 breaths. **Recite a Scripture verse.**

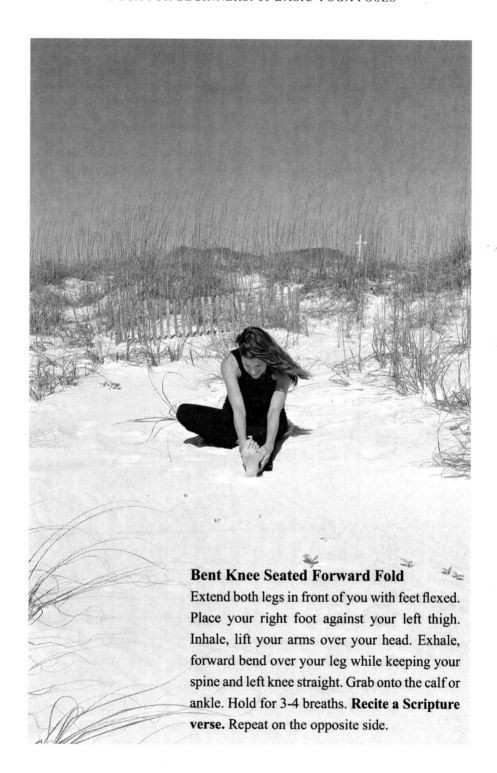

Bent Knee Seated Forward Fold
Extend both legs in front of you with feet flexed. Place your right foot against your left thigh. Inhale, lift your arms over your head. Exhale, forward bend over your leg while keeping your spine and left knee straight. Grab onto the calf or ankle. Hold for 3-4 breaths. **Recite a Scripture verse.** Repeat on the opposite side.

61

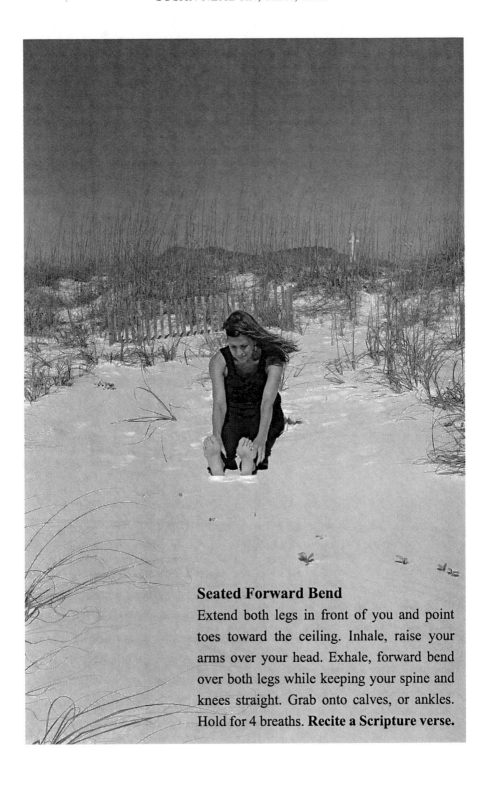

Seated Forward Bend
Extend both legs in front of you and point toes toward the ceiling. Inhale, raise your arms over your head. Exhale, forward bend over both legs while keeping your spine and knees straight. Grab onto calves, or ankles. Hold for 4 breaths. **Recite a Scripture verse.**

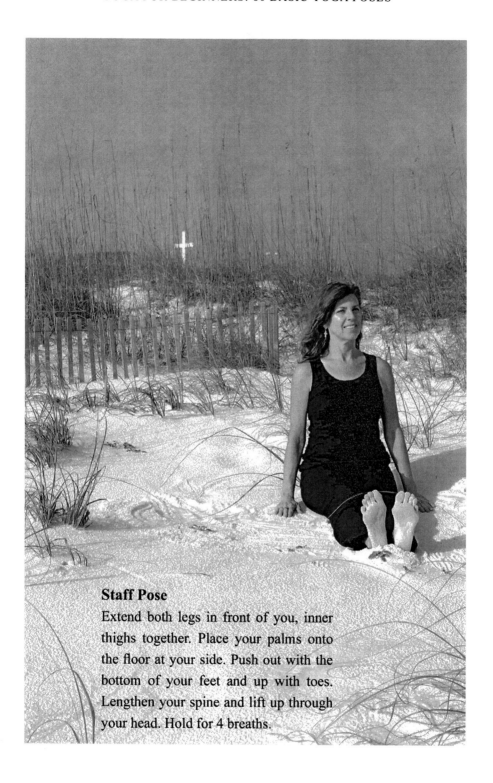

Staff Pose
Extend both legs in front of you, inner thighs together. Place your palms onto the floor at your side. Push out with the bottom of your feet and up with toes. Lengthen your spine and lift up through your head. Hold for 4 breaths.

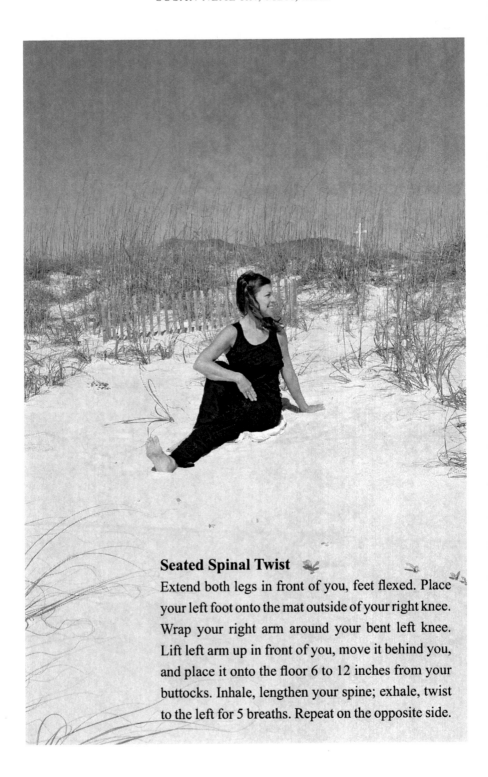

Seated Spinal Twist

Extend both legs in front of you, feet flexed. Place your left foot onto the mat outside of your right knee. Wrap your right arm around your bent left knee. Lift left arm up in front of you, move it behind you, and place it onto the floor 6 to 12 inches from your buttocks. Inhale, lengthen your spine; exhale, twist to the left for 5 breaths. Repeat on the opposite side.

Chapter 10

KNEELING POSES

Now, we will get onto our hands and knees for our kneeling postures. First, we will begin with the Lion pose because it is essential to stretch all the muscles in our face, as well as the rest of our bodies.

Yoga Posture Modification Suggestions

Downward Dog-move into the Half Dog where you stay on your knees and forearms while lifting your tailbone up.

Camel-from a kneeling position, sit on your heels and place your palms flat on the floor behind you with fingertips pointed away from your body. Lift your pelvis so you have a straight line between your knees, neck, and head.

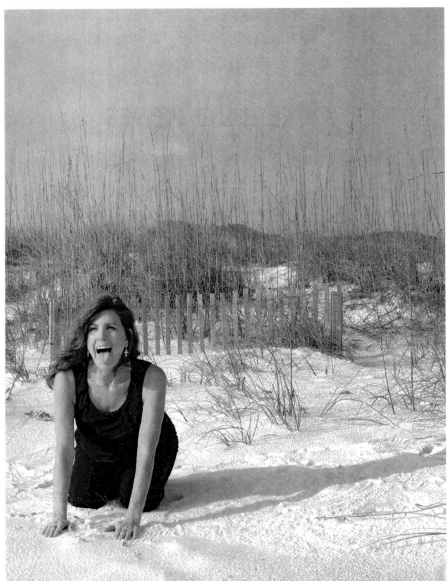

Lion

It is important to stretch the muscles in your face as well as the rest of your body. Sit on your heels, spread your hands and place them onto the floor in front of you. Open your mouth, extend tongue, widen eyes, and stretch all the muscles in your face. Hold for 4-6 breaths, and then roar like God's mighty Lion of Judah!

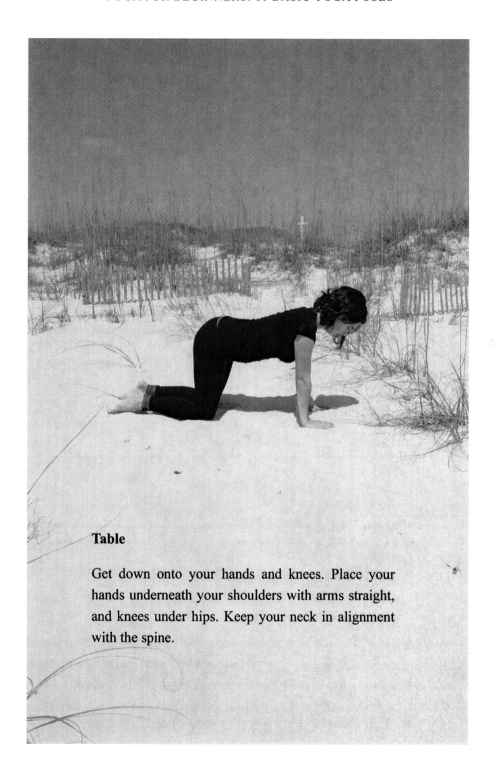

Table

Get down onto your hands and knees. Place your hands underneath your shoulders with arms straight, and knees under hips. Keep your neck in alignment with the spine.

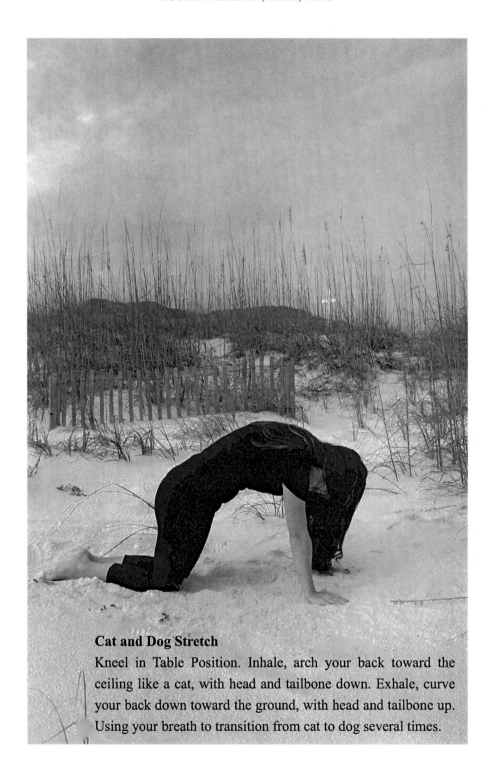

Cat and Dog Stretch
Kneel in Table Position. Inhale, arch your back toward the ceiling like a cat, with head and tailbone down. Exhale, curve your back down toward the ground, with head and tailbone up. Using your breath to transition from cat to dog several times.

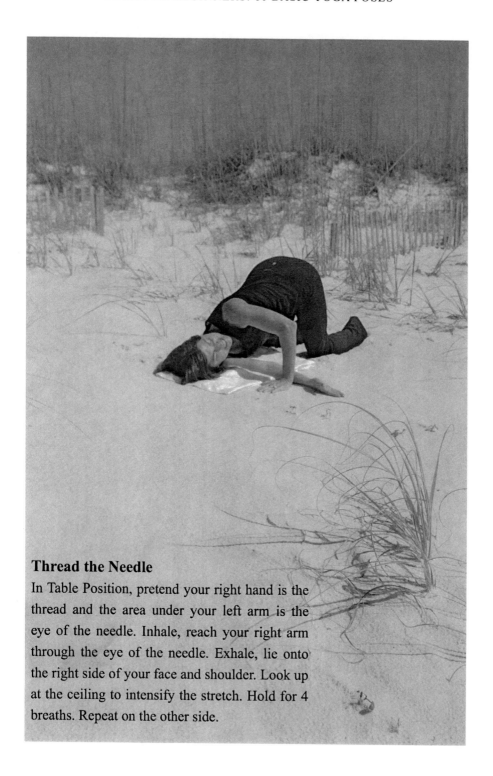

Thread the Needle

In Table Position, pretend your right hand is the thread and the area under your left arm is the eye of the needle. Inhale, reach your right arm through the eye of the needle. Exhale, lie onto the right side of your face and shoulder. Look up at the ceiling to intensify the stretch. Hold for 4 breaths. Repeat on the other side.

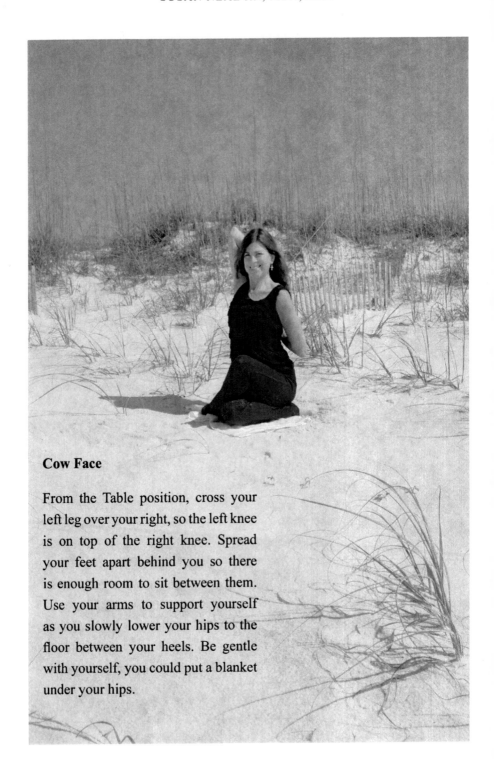

Cow Face

From the Table position, cross your left leg over your right, so the left knee is on top of the right knee. Spread your feet apart behind you so there is enough room to sit between them. Use your arms to support yourself as you slowly lower your hips to the floor between your heels. Be gentle with yourself, you could put a blanket under your hips.

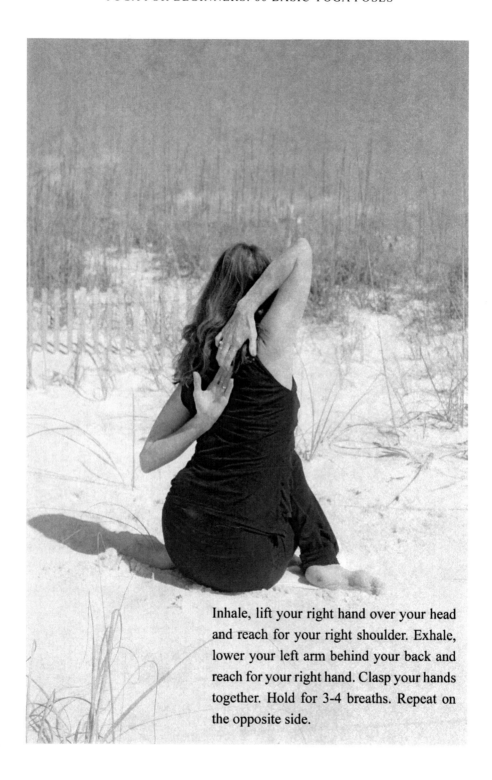

Inhale, lift your right hand over your head and reach for your right shoulder. Exhale, lower your left arm behind your back and reach for your right hand. Clasp your hands together. Hold for 3-4 breaths. Repeat on the opposite side.

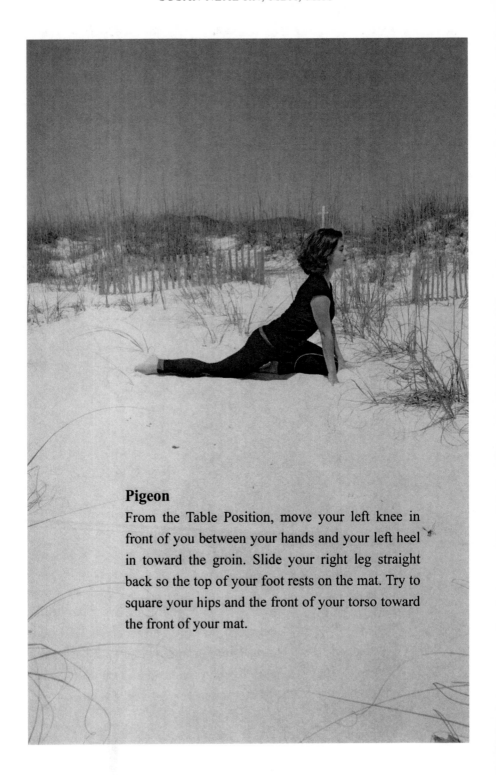

Pigeon

From the Table Position, move your left knee in front of you between your hands and your left heel in toward the groin. Slide your right leg straight back so the top of your foot rests on the mat. Try to square your hips and the front of your torso toward the front of your mat.

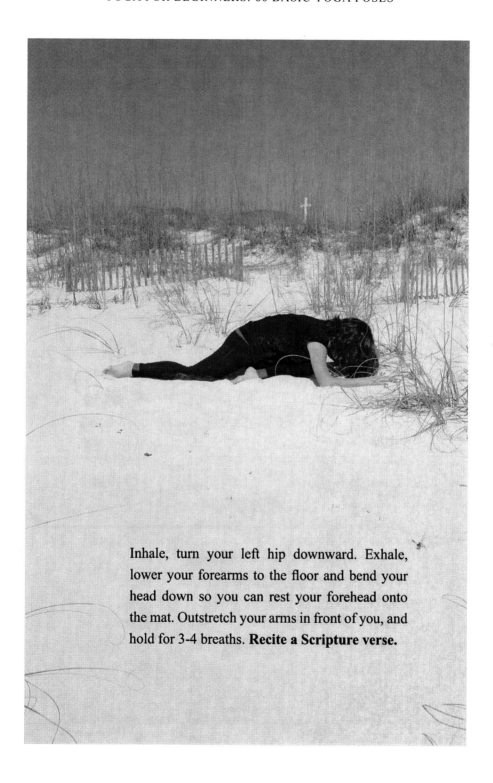

Inhale, turn your left hip downward. Exhale, lower your forearms to the floor and bend your head down so you can rest your forehead onto the mat. Outstretch your arms in front of you, and hold for 3-4 breaths. **Recite a Scripture verse.**

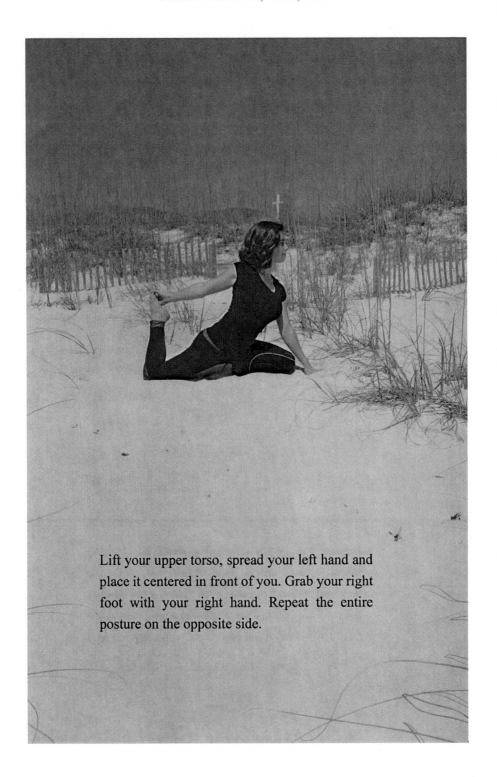

Lift your upper torso, spread your left hand and place it centered in front of you. Grab your right foot with your right hand. Repeat the entire posture on the opposite side.

Downward Dog

From Table position, curl your toes into the floor. Exhale, lift your bottom up toward the ceiling. Straighten your elbows and back while keeping your neck in alignment with the spine. Press your chest toward your knees.

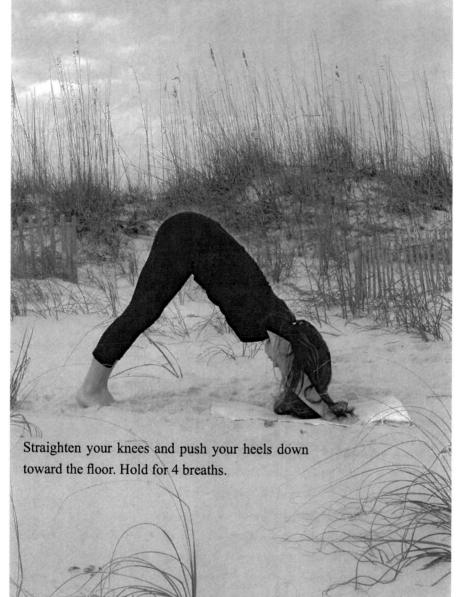

Straighten your knees and push your heels down toward the floor. Hold for 4 breaths.

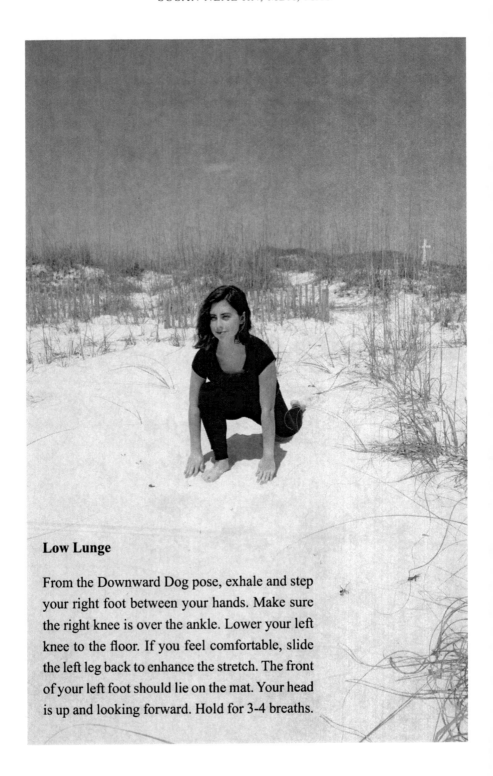

Low Lunge

From the Downward Dog pose, exhale and step your right foot between your hands. Make sure the right knee is over the ankle. Lower your left knee to the floor. If you feel comfortable, slide the left leg back to enhance the stretch. The front of your left foot should lie on the mat. Your head is up and looking forward. Hold for 3-4 breaths.

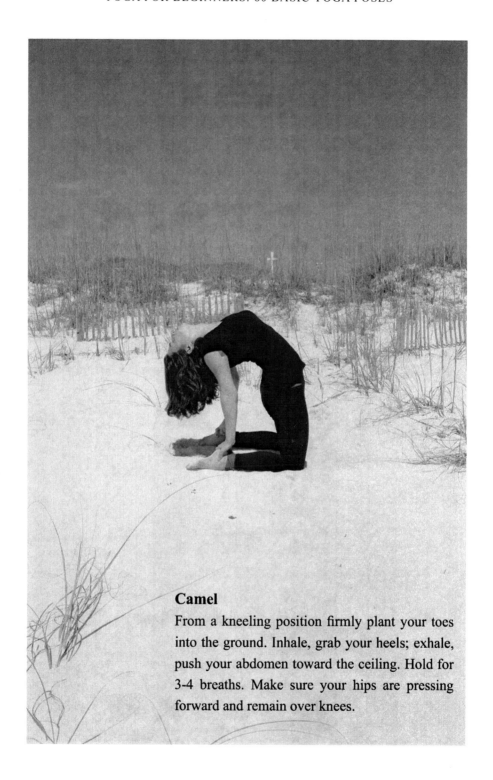

Camel

From a kneeling position firmly plant your toes into the ground. Inhale, grab your heels; exhale, push your abdomen toward the ceiling. Hold for 3-4 breaths. Make sure your hips are pressing forward and remain over knees.

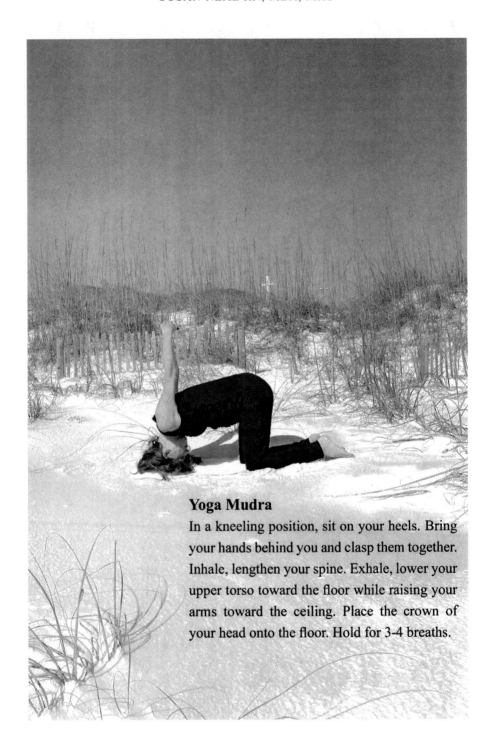

Yoga Mudra

In a kneeling position, sit on your heels. Bring your hands behind you and clasp them together. Inhale, lengthen your spine. Exhale, lower your upper torso toward the floor while raising your arms toward the ceiling. Place the crown of your head onto the floor. Hold for 3-4 breaths.

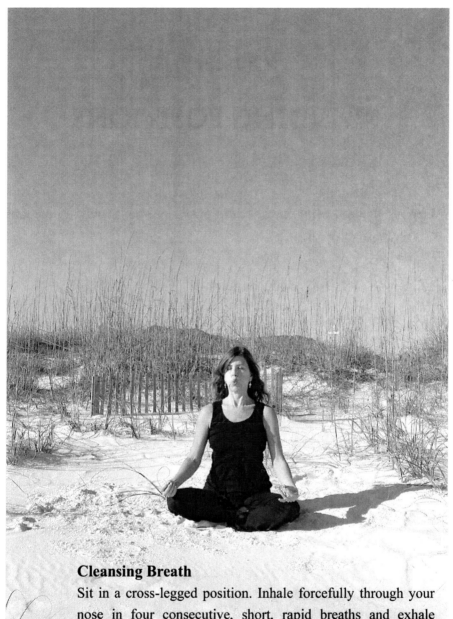

Cleansing Breath
Sit in a cross-legged position. Inhale forcefully through your nose in four consecutive, short, rapid breaths and exhale forcefully once through your mouth. Repeat this sequence 10-12 times.

Chapter 11

STANDING POSITIONS

We will transition from our kneeling poses into our standing positions by moving into the squat.

Yoga Posture Modification Suggestions

Dancer-stand in front of a wall so your fingertips touch the wall as you lean forward into the pose.

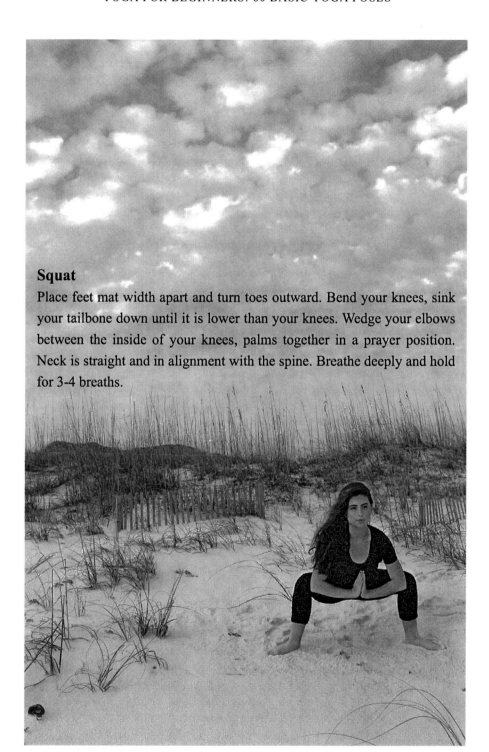

Squat

Place feet mat width apart and turn toes outward. Bend your knees, sink your tailbone down until it is lower than your knees. Wedge your elbows between the inside of your knees, palms together in a prayer position. Neck is straight and in alignment with the spine. Breathe deeply and hold for 3-4 breaths.

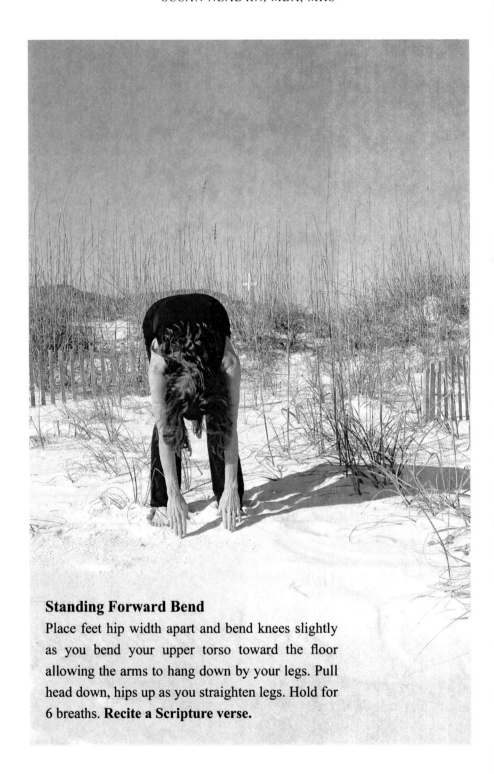

Standing Forward Bend

Place feet hip width apart and bend knees slightly as you bend your upper torso toward the floor allowing the arms to hang down by your legs. Pull head down, hips up as you straighten legs. Hold for 6 breaths. **Recite a Scripture verse.**

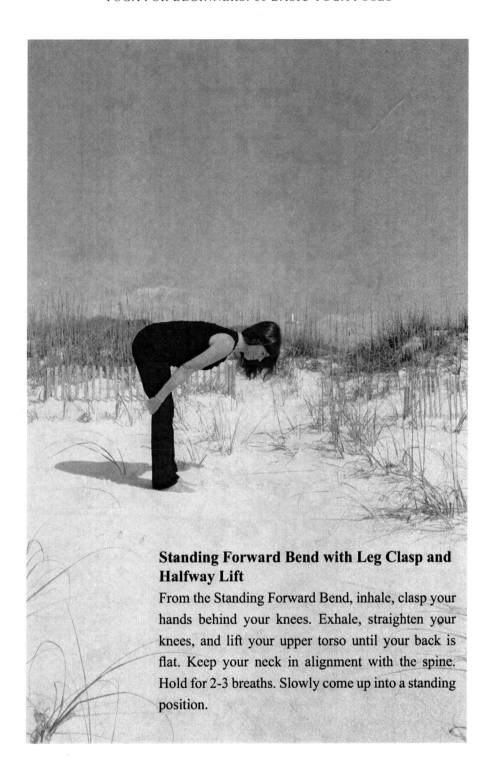

Standing Forward Bend with Leg Clasp and Halfway Lift

From the Standing Forward Bend, inhale, clasp your hands behind your knees. Exhale, straighten your knees, and lift your upper torso until your back is flat. Keep your neck in alignment with the spine. Hold for 2-3 breaths. Slowly come up into a standing position.

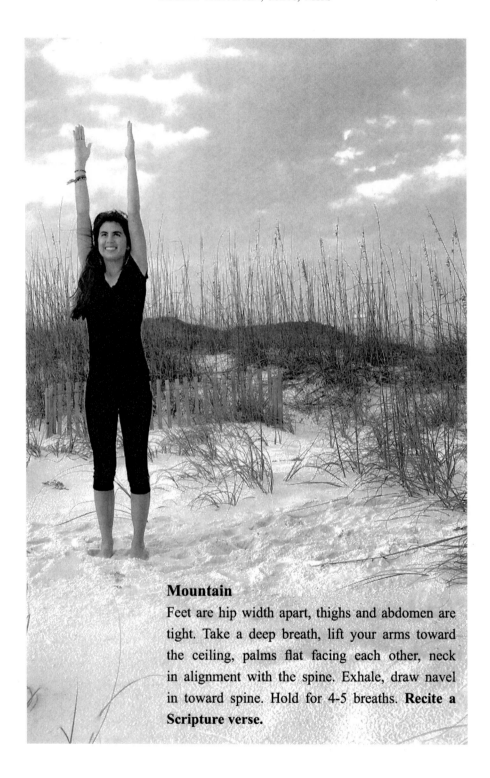

Mountain

Feet are hip width apart, thighs and abdomen are tight. Take a deep breath, lift your arms toward the ceiling, palms flat facing each other, neck in alignment with the spine. Exhale, draw navel in toward spine. Hold for 4-5 breaths. **Recite a Scripture verse.**

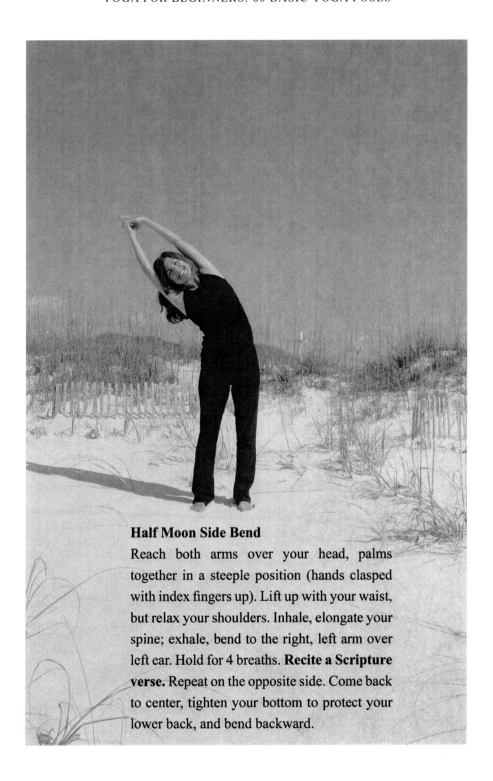

Half Moon Side Bend
Reach both arms over your head, palms together in a steeple position (hands clasped with index fingers up). Lift up with your waist, but relax your shoulders. Inhale, elongate your spine; exhale, bend to the right, left arm over left ear. Hold for 4 breaths. **Recite a Scripture verse.** Repeat on the opposite side. Come back to center, tighten your bottom to protect your lower back, and bend backward.

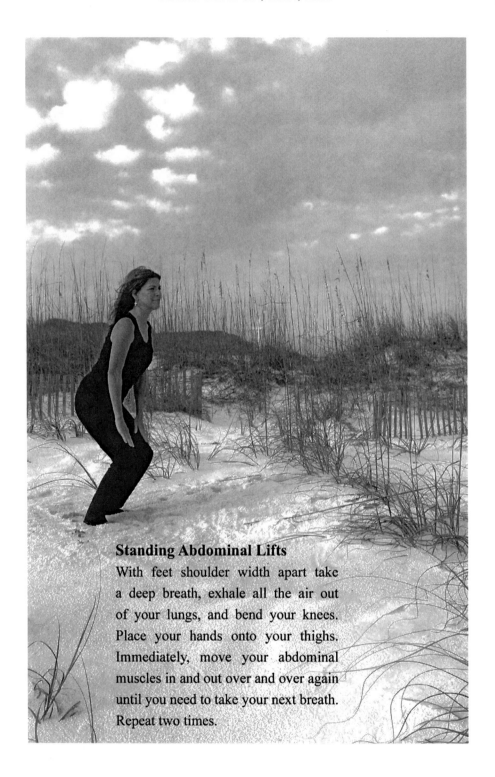

Standing Abdominal Lifts
With feet shoulder width apart take
a deep breath, exhale all the air out
of your lungs, and bend your knees.
Place your hands onto your thighs.
Immediately, move your abdominal
muscles in and out over and over again
until you need to take your next breath.
Repeat two times.

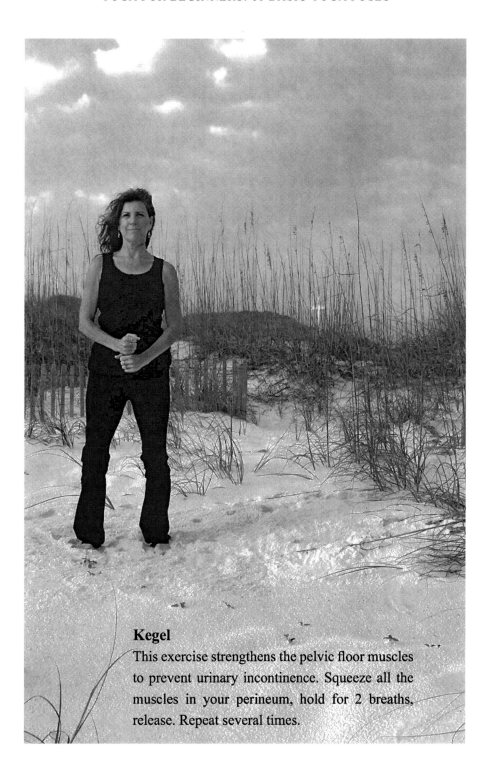

Kegel
This exercise strengthens the pelvic floor muscles to prevent urinary incontinence. Squeeze all the muscles in your perineum, hold for 2 breaths, release. Repeat several times.

Warrior I

Take a large step forward with your right foot. Make sure your right knee is over your ankle. Press the left heel toward the floor and keep this leg straight.

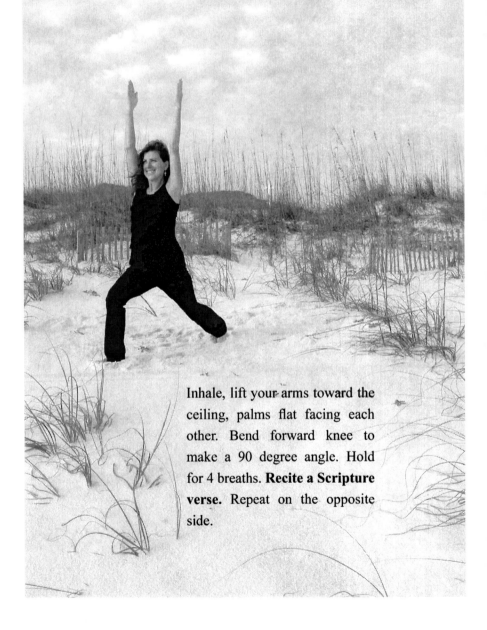

Inhale, lift your arms toward the ceiling, palms flat facing each other. Bend forward knee to make a 90 degree angle. Hold for 4 breaths. **Recite a Scripture verse.** Repeat on the opposite side.

Warrior II

Take a large step to the side with your left foot. Pivot your left foot so toes are pointed to the left, and right foot is at a 45-degree angle. Inhale, raise arms into a T position, palms down and look at your left hand. Exhale, bend left knee and lunge with straight right leg. Make sure left knee is over your ankle and not the toes.

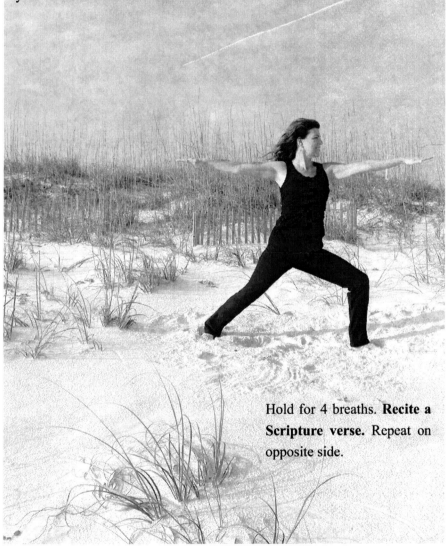

Hold for 4 breaths. **Recite a Scripture verse.** Repeat on opposite side.

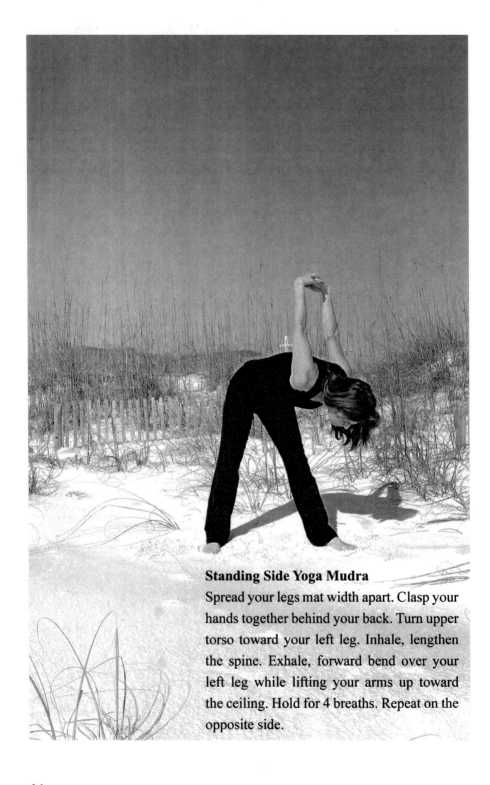

Standing Side Yoga Mudra

Spread your legs mat width apart. Clasp your hands together behind your back. Turn upper torso toward your left leg. Inhale, lengthen the spine. Exhale, forward bend over your left leg while lifting your arms up toward the ceiling. Hold for 4 breaths. Repeat on the opposite side.

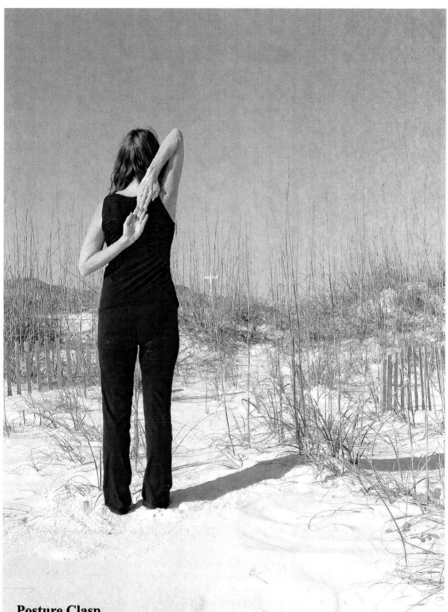

Posture Clasp

Inhale, lift your right hand over your head and reach for your right shoulder. Exhale, lower your left arm behind your back and reach for your right hand. Clasp your hands together, and move the left arm up and right down. Hold for 3-4 breaths. Repeat on the opposite side.

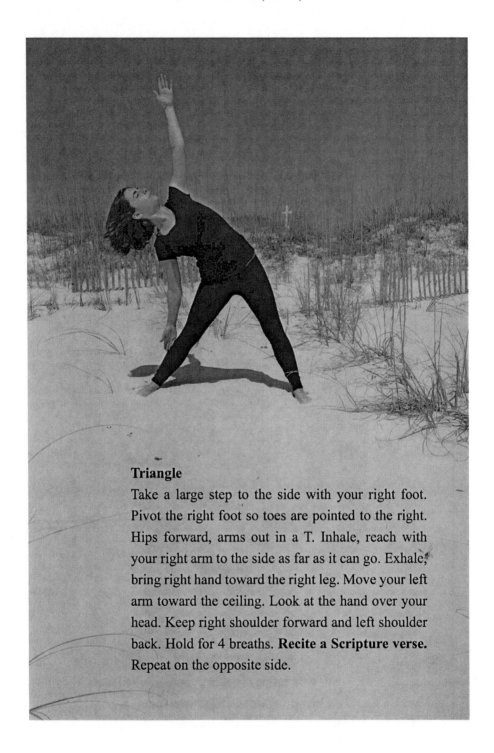

Triangle

Take a large step to the side with your right foot. Pivot the right foot so toes are pointed to the right. Hips forward, arms out in a T. Inhale, reach with your right arm to the side as far as it can go. Exhale, bring right hand toward the right leg. Move your left arm toward the ceiling. Look at the hand over your head. Keep right shoulder forward and left shoulder back. Hold for 4 breaths. **Recite a Scripture verse.** Repeat on the opposite side.

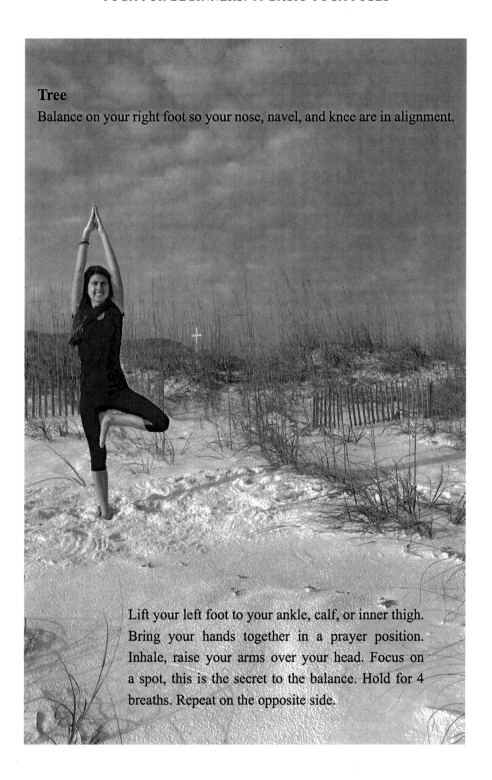

Tree
Balance on your right foot so your nose, navel, and knee are in alignment.

Lift your left foot to your ankle, calf, or inner thigh. Bring your hands together in a prayer position. Inhale, raise your arms over your head. Focus on a spot, this is the secret to the balance. Hold for 4 breaths. Repeat on the opposite side.

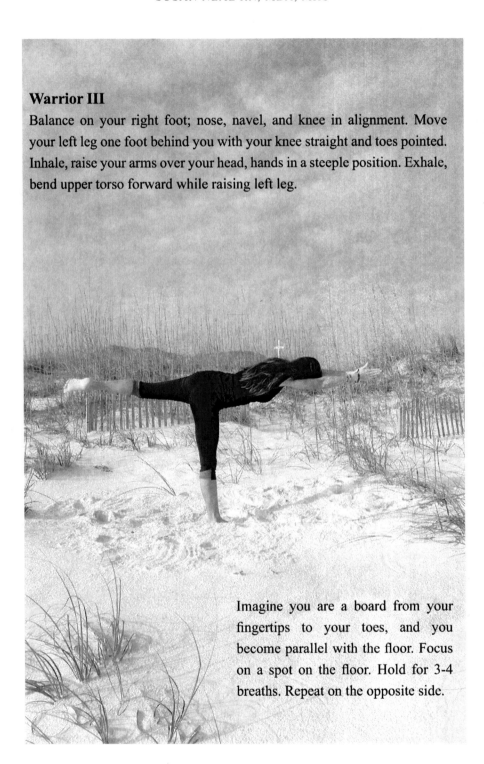

Warrior III

Balance on your right foot; nose, navel, and knee in alignment. Move your left leg one foot behind you with your knee straight and toes pointed. Inhale, raise your arms over your head, hands in a steeple position. Exhale, bend upper torso forward while raising left leg.

Imagine you are a board from your fingertips to your toes, and you become parallel with the floor. Focus on a spot on the floor. Hold for 3-4 breaths. Repeat on the opposite side.

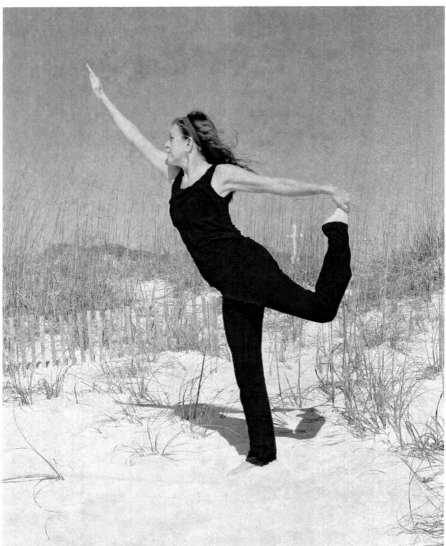

Dancer

Balance on your right foot. Inhale, raise your right arm, elbow straight, over your head with fingertips pointed. Exhale, lift left foot behind you and grab it with your left hand. Lean forward with your upper body while pulling your left leg back behind you. Hold for 3-4 breaths. Repeat on the opposite side.

Chapter 12

PRONE (BELLY DOWN) YOGA POSTURES

Now that we have completed our standing postures we will lie down onto our abdomen for our belly down poses.

Yoga Posture Modification Suggestions

Cobra-keep your forearms on the mat while moving your upper torso up. This modified Cobra is called the Sphinx pose.

Plank-keep your forearms on the mat when moving into the Plank. This decreases the pressure on your wrists

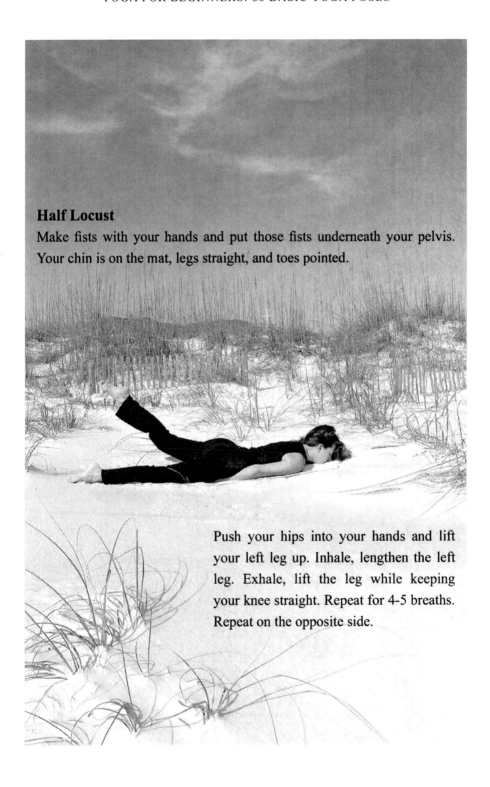

Half Locust

Make fists with your hands and put those fists underneath your pelvis. Your chin is on the mat, legs straight, and toes pointed.

Push your hips into your hands and lift your left leg up. Inhale, lengthen the left leg. Exhale, lift the leg while keeping your knee straight. Repeat for 4-5 breaths. Repeat on the opposite side.

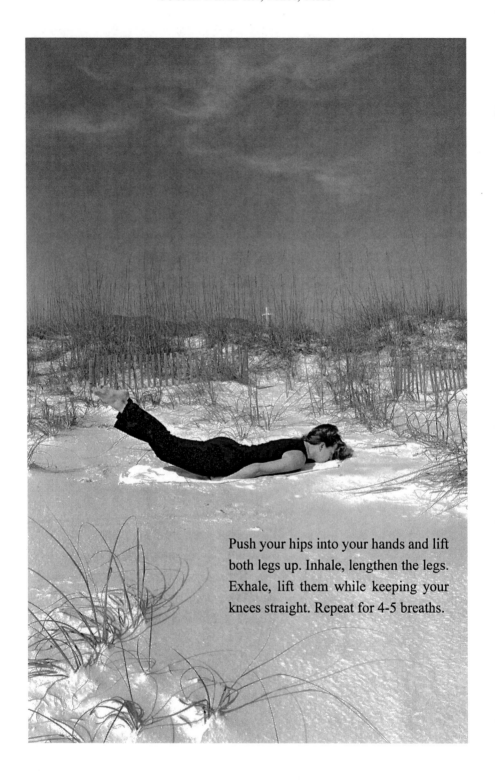

Push your hips into your hands and lift both legs up. Inhale, lengthen the legs. Exhale, lift them while keeping your knees straight. Repeat for 4-5 breaths.

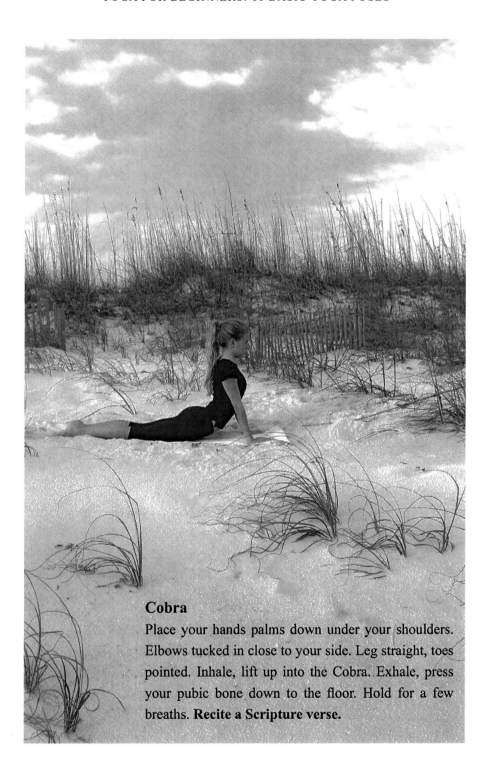

Cobra

Place your hands palms down under your shoulders.
Elbows tucked in close to your side. Leg straight, toes
pointed. Inhale, lift up into the Cobra. Exhale, press
your pubic bone down to the floor. Hold for a few
breaths. **Recite a Scripture verse.**

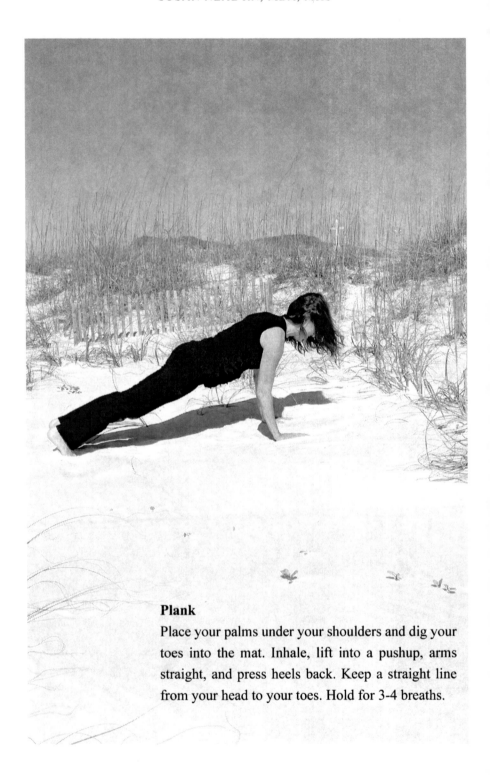

Plank

Place your palms under your shoulders and dig your toes into the mat. Inhale, lift into a pushup, arms straight, and press heels back. Keep a straight line from your head to your toes. Hold for 3-4 breaths.

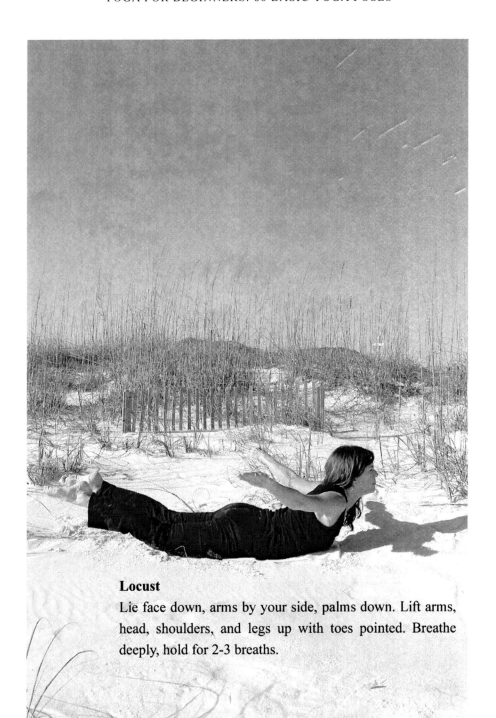

Locust
Lie face down, arms by your side, palms down. Lift arms, head, shoulders, and legs up with toes pointed. Breathe deeply, hold for 2-3 breaths.

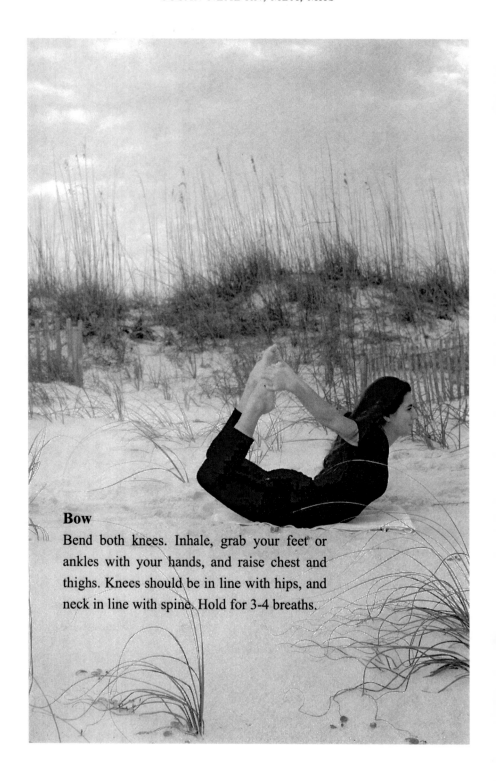

Bow

Bend both knees. Inhale, grab your feet or ankles with your hands, and raise chest and thighs. Knees should be in line with hips, and neck in line with spine. Hold for 3-4 breaths.

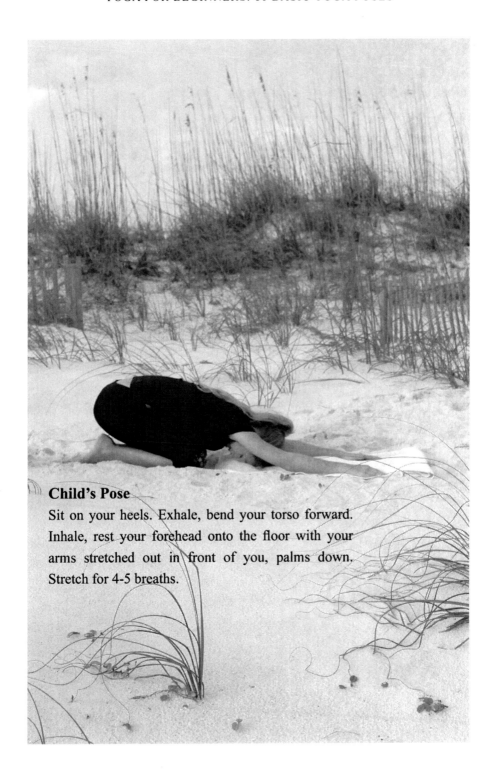

Child's Pose

Sit on your heels. Exhale, bend your torso forward. Inhale, rest your forehead onto the floor with your arms stretched out in front of you, palms down. Stretch for 4-5 breaths.

Chapter 13

SUPINE (BACK DOWN) YOGA POSTURES

Get up and lie down onto your back for the back down postures.

Yoga Posture Modification Suggestions

Bridge-stay in the basic pose of the Bridge, therefore, you do not clasp your hands together under your back.

Shoulder Stand-only lift your legs up into the air, not your pelvis. Then perform the ankle movements.

Fish-do not tilt your head back, instead stay in the basic posture of the Fish with your upper torso weight on your elbows.

Double Leg Raises

Lie on your back with your arms by your side. Raise both legs toward the ceiling. Keep your knees straight and buttocks on the mat. Slowly, lower your legs toward the floor and at the same time push your lower back down toward the floor.

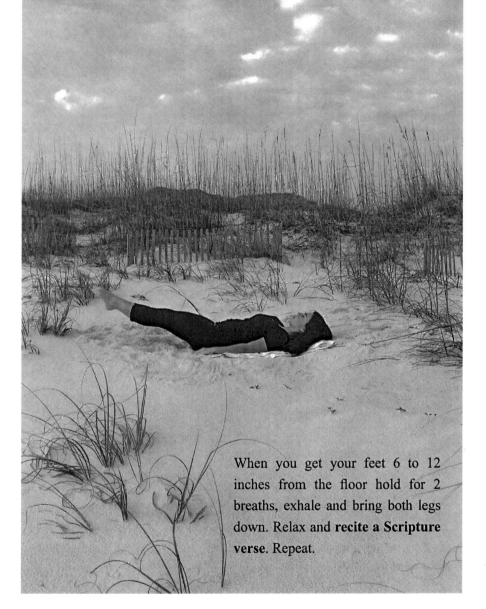

When you get your feet 6 to 12 inches from the floor hold for 2 breaths, exhale and bring both legs down. Relax and **recite a Scripture verse**. Repeat.

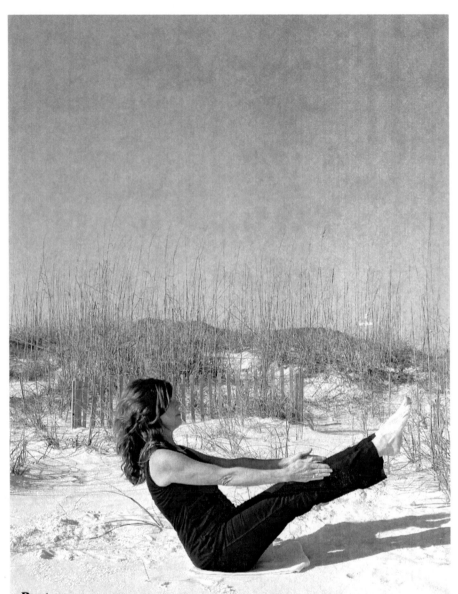

Boat

From a seated position, inhale, bend the knees; exhale, lift both legs up.
Lean back, keep your neck in alignment with the spine. Straighten your
legs and balance on your sits bone. Lift arms, elbows straight, so hands are
by your knees. Hold for 3-4 breaths.

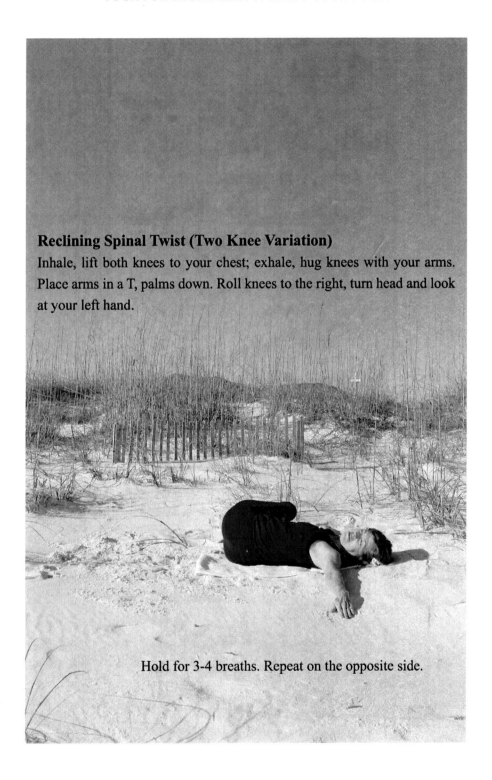

Reclining Spinal Twist (Two Knee Variation)
Inhale, lift both knees to your chest; exhale, hug knees with your arms.
Place arms in a T, palms down. Roll knees to the right, turn head and look
at your left hand.

Hold for 3-4 breaths. Repeat on the opposite side.

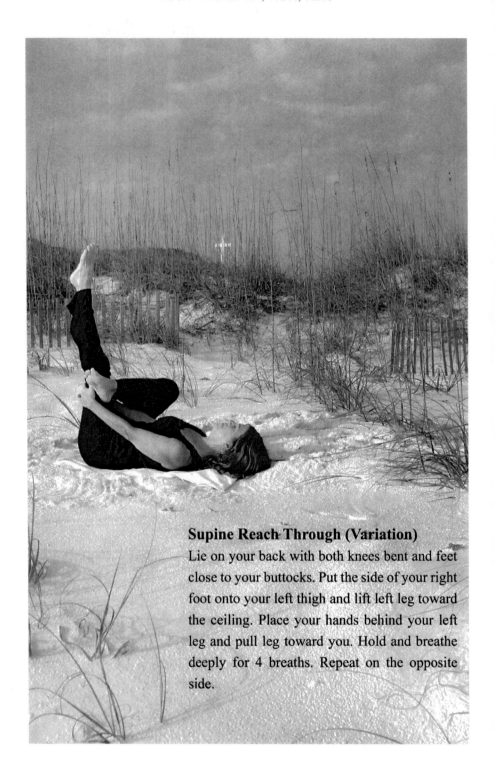

Supine Reach Through (Variation)
Lie on your back with both knees bent and feet close to your buttocks. Put the side of your right foot onto your left thigh and lift left leg toward the ceiling. Place your hands behind your left leg and pull leg toward you. Hold and breathe deeply for 4 breaths. Repeat on the opposite side.

Bridge

Lie on your back with knees bent, feet close to your buttocks, and arms by your side, so fingertips touch heels. Inhale, firmly press feet into the mat. Exhale, lift your pelvis toward the ceiling so you are a straight line between your chest and pelvis. Distribute weight evenly between feet and shoulders. This is the basic posture of the bridge.

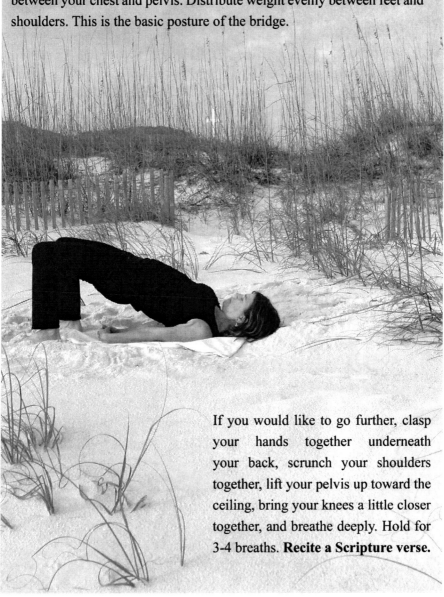

If you would like to go further, clasp your hands together underneath your back, scrunch your shoulders together, lift your pelvis up toward the ceiling, bring your knees a little closer together, and breathe deeply. Hold for 3-4 breaths. **Recite a Scripture verse.**

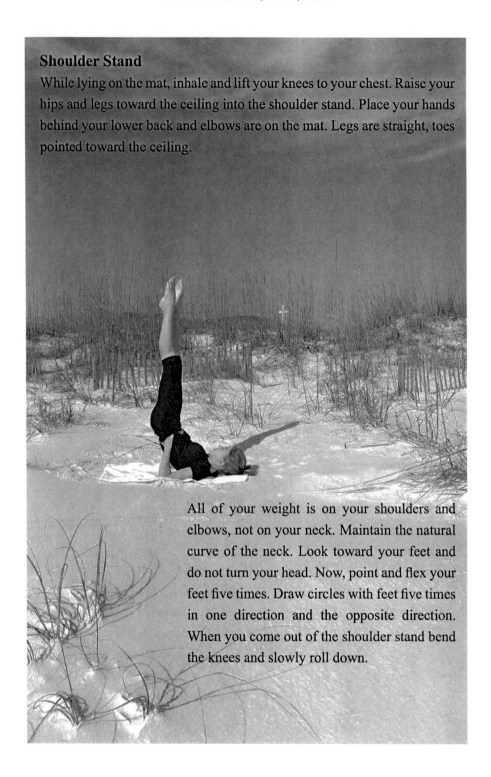

Shoulder Stand
While lying on the mat, inhale and lift your knees to your chest. Raise your hips and legs toward the ceiling into the shoulder stand. Place your hands behind your lower back and elbows are on the mat. Legs are straight, toes pointed toward the ceiling.

All of your weight is on your shoulders and elbows, not on your neck. Maintain the natural curve of the neck. Look toward your feet and do not turn your head. Now, point and flex your feet five times. Draw circles with feet five times in one direction and the opposite direction. When you come out of the shoulder stand bend the knees and slowly roll down.

Fish

While lying on your mat, make a diamond shape with your hands by touching index fingers and thumbs. Tuck hands, palms down, underneath your buttocks so the tailbone sits between your thumbs and index fingers. Legs are straight and together.

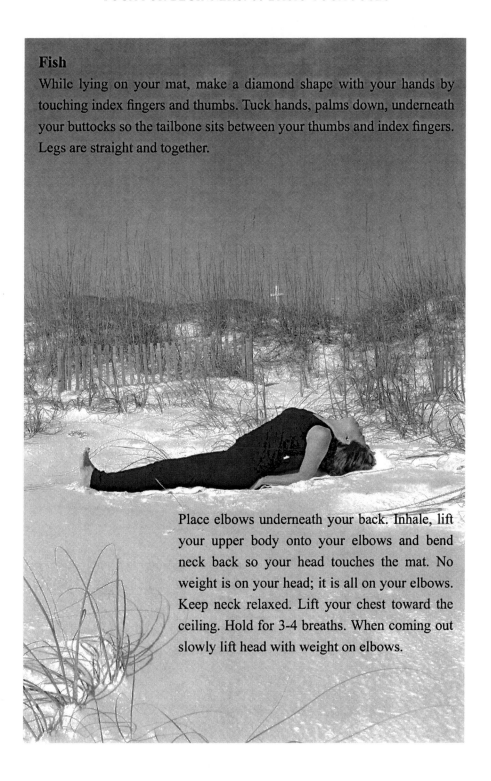

Place elbows underneath your back. Inhale, lift your upper body onto your elbows and bend neck back so your head touches the mat. No weight is on your head; it is all on your elbows. Keep neck relaxed. Lift your chest toward the ceiling. Hold for 3-4 breaths. When coming out slowly lift head with weight on elbows.

Lying Spinal Twist (One Leg Variation)

Lie on your back with your arms out in a T. Inhale, put your left foot on top of your right knee. Exhale, roll your left knee toward your right hand, twisting the spine.

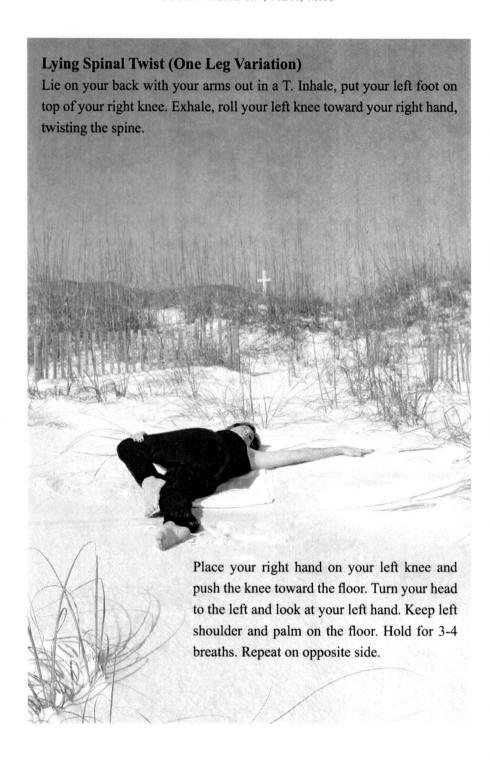

Place your right hand on your left knee and push the knee toward the floor. Turn your head to the left and look at your left hand. Keep left shoulder and palm on the floor. Hold for 3-4 breaths. Repeat on opposite side.

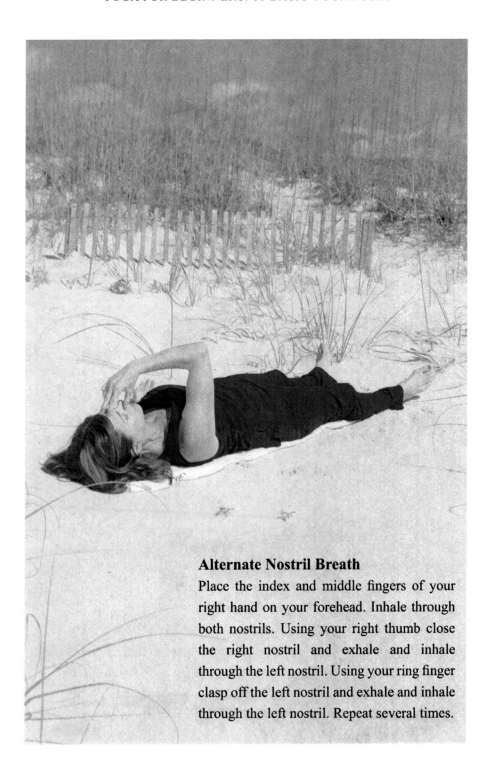

Alternate Nostril Breath
Place the index and middle fingers of your right hand on your forehead. Inhale through both nostrils. Using your right thumb close the right nostril and exhale and inhale through the left nostril. Using your ring finger clasp off the left nostril and exhale and inhale through the left nostril. Repeat several times.

Chapter 14

RELAXATION

Relaxation is an important component of the yoga class. Relaxing your body prepares your mind for the meditative session at the end. We will begin relaxation in the Corpse pose.

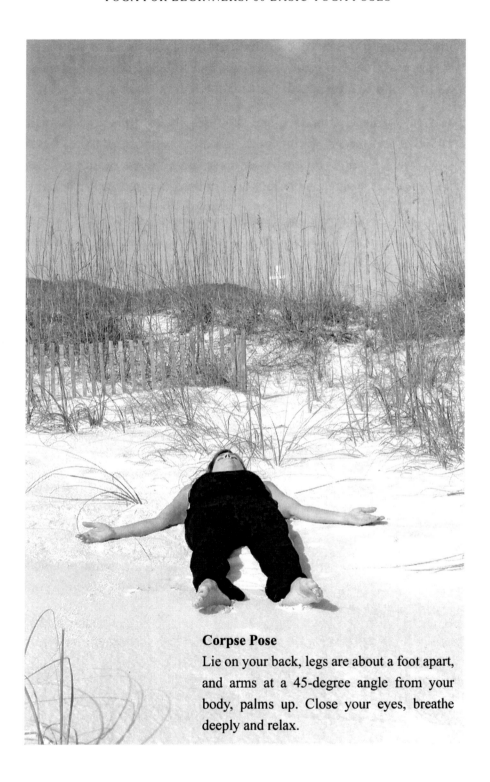

Corpse Pose
Lie on your back, legs are about a foot apart, and arms at a 45-degree angle from your body, palms up. Close your eyes, breathe deeply and relax.

You are going to relax your entire body from your head to your toes. Begin by relaxing your head. Relax each hair follicle from your forehead to the crown of your head, all the way down to the base of your neck.

Loosen your neck, shoulders, and shoulder blades. Relax the thoracic vertebra in the center of your back and all your muscles there. Relax your lumbar vertebra in your lower back and all those muscles. Relax your buttocks, sacrum, and tailbone. Your back is completely relaxed.

Now you will relax your face. Begin by releasing any tension in your forehead, eyes, and nose. Loosen your cheeks, ears, and jaw line all the way to your chin. Relax your lips. Swallow, relax your throat. Relax your neck from your chin all the way down your neck to your shoulders.

Release tension in your shoulders and upper arms all the way to your elbows. Relax your forearms, wrists, and hands. Allowing the tension to flow out through your fingertips.

Take a deep breath and know that your heart and lungs are functioning perfectly. Loosen your chest and abdominal muscles, all the way to your pelvis. Relax your intestinal organs, and the organs in your pelvis. Relax your pelvis.

Release the tension in your hips and thighs. The relaxation moves all the way down to the knees, calves, ankles, into the heels, up the feet, and out the toes.

Your body is completely at ease. You are lying in the palm of God's hand. You do not have a care in the world because you give all your cares to God.

Recite a Scripture verse — recite either the last verse in the lesson or the primary verse that you repeated throughout the class.

You are lying in the palm of God's hand, spend some time with him, and I will tell you when to get up in a few minutes.

Five minutes later: On the count of three you will become awake, alert, and energized. One, open your eyes and become aware of your surroundings. Two, wiggle your fingers and toes. Three, reach your arms over your head and stretch from your head to your toes.

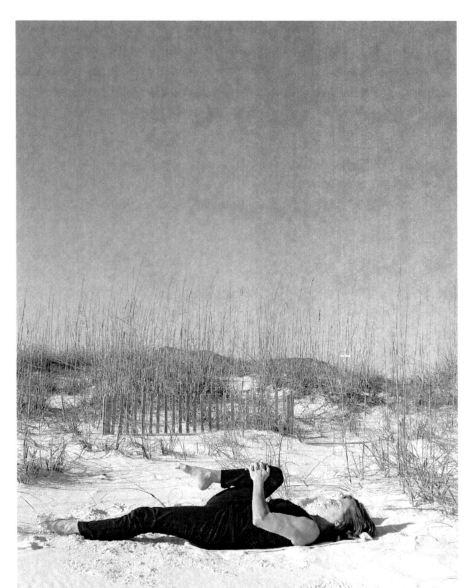

Single Knee Hug

While lying on your back with both legs straight, inhale, bend your right knee up to your chest. Exhale, wrap your arms around the knee and squeeze it to your chest. Repeat on the opposite side.

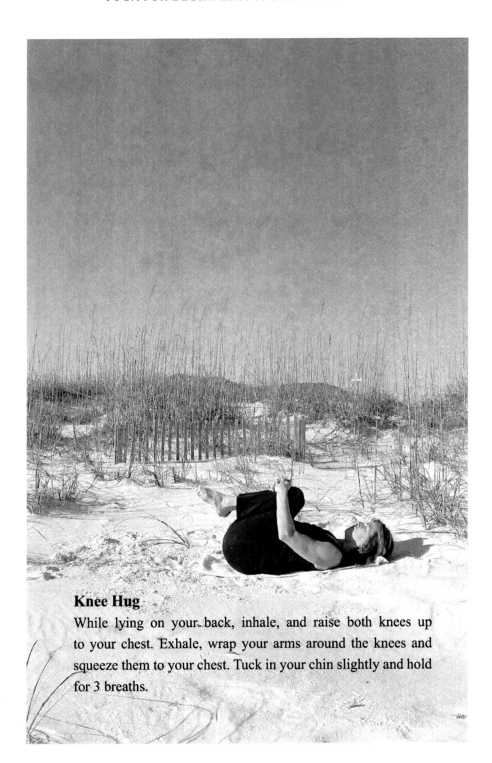

Knee Hug

While lying on your back, inhale, and raise both knees up
to your chest. Exhale, wrap your arms around the knees and
squeeze them to your chest. Tuck in your chin slightly and hold
for 3 breaths.

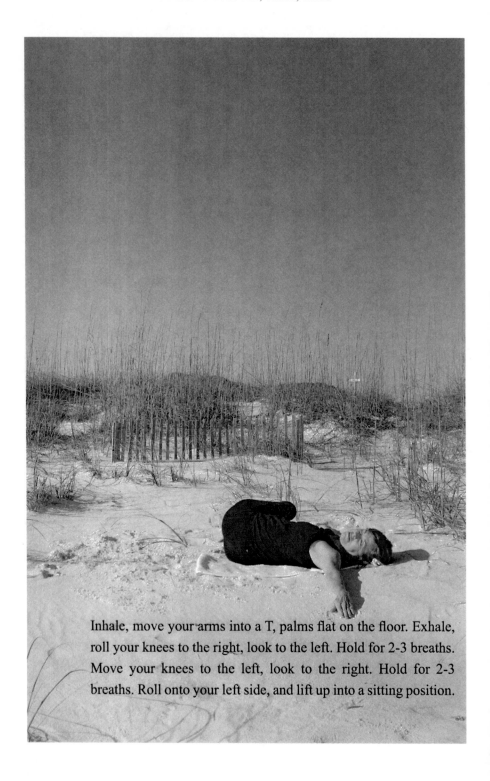

Inhale, move your arms into a T, palms flat on the floor. Exhale, roll your knees to the right, look to the left. Hold for 2-3 breaths. Move your knees to the left, look to the right. Hold for 2-3 breaths. Roll onto your left side, and lift up into a sitting position.

Chapter 15

EAT TO LIVE

I weigh the same in my mid-fifties as I did in my early twenties because I research and evaluate everything I eat. If it is from a bag or a box, it is dead food and I try not to eat it. Have you heard the saying "shelf life means no life?"

The following healthy eating guidelines are my secret to maintaining optimal weight and brain health. This low-carbohydrate, low-glycemic, anti-inflammatory diet is the type of diet recommended for improving memory and cognition. No more brain fog!

In fact, this is the same type of diet used in a research study published June 2016 by Dale E. Bredesen. The article, "Reversal of Cognitive Decline in Alzheimer's Disease," is the first clinical study where Alzheimer's symptoms improved. In this study, a patient who had well-documented Alzheimer's disease was on the program for 22 months which resulted in his neuropsychological testing improving 81% from the 3rd percentile to the 84th. Finally, there is hope for these devastating diseases of the brain!

Obtain a summary of this therapeutic program which includes a list of 24 things you can do to improve your memory and prevent or reverse Alzheimer's Disease and dementia. Purchase the summary at this link http://christianyoga.com/dvd-products.

A low glycemic diet does not raise your blood sugar and insulin levels. Foods high in carbohydrates cause a release of glucose into the bloodstream and a corresponding rise in insulin. The following are high-carbohydrate foods that should be avoided: cakes, crackers, sugary cereals and drinks, flours, bread products, jellies/jams, and refined potato products.

The following diet minimizes the high blood sugar spikes.

- About 50% of my food is fresh organic vegetables.

- Eat one-two servings of fresh, raw fruit per day. Low glycemic fruits include green apples, berries, cherries, pears, plums, and grapefruit.

- Do not always eat cooked foods. Eat a couple of servings of RAW fruits and vegetables every day. I eat a salad for lunch with either nuts or some meat. When eating out, I order a salad and coleslaw as my sides since both are raw.

- Have 25% of your food be an animal or vegetable protein such as beans, nuts, and lean meats. Fish is especially nutritious.

- A variety of different nuts and seeds are excellent sources of protein, minerals, and essential fatty acids.

- Avoid everything white—sugar, flour, rice, pasta, and bread. Instead, eat more fruits, vegetables, and low-glycemic grains such as quinoa and pearled barley.

- Do not eat sugary cereals. Instead, eat oatmeal, fruit, or granola (but watch the sugar: it can be extremely high).

- Do not eat wheat. Dr. William Davis, author of *Wheat Belly* states, "Whole wheat bread increases blood sugar as much as or more than table sugar." He placed his overweight, diabetic-prone patients on a low-glycemic whole foods diet which excluded wheat, for three months. Results included:

-Diabetics became non-diabetics

-Acid reflux disappeared

-Irritable bowel syndrome went away

-Rheumatoid arthritis pain decreased

-Asthma symptoms improved or resolved completely

-Rashes disappeared

-Energy increased

-Lost weight

-Experienced clearer thinking and greater focus

- If you are still having digestive issues after you have eliminated wheat, take a digestive enzyme with meals. Anyone over 40 will benefit from them as we all experience a decrease in gastric enzymes with age. I have also found *The Eat Right 4 Your Type* by Dr. Peter D'Adamo to be very helpful in figuring out what foods to avoid so you do not have digestive problems and to make sure your blood does not agglutinate.

- Chew your food thoroughly because this is where digestion begins.

- Try not to eat anything that contains more than 10 g of sugar in one serving.

- Eat non-traditional grains such as quinoa, amaranth, pearled barley, and oats.

- Eat cultured foods such as Kimchi, sauerkraut, and cultured plain Greek yogurt because they are loaded with natural probiotics. Add 1-2 tablespoons to a meal a couple of times a week or eat the yogurt as a snack. Personally, I take a good probiotic capsule every day.

- Do not drink with meals because this dilutes your digestive enzymes which are secreted to break down the food in your stomach.

- Drink eight glasses of water every day. Other than coffee or tea, water should be your only beverage, and these beverages should not count toward the eight glasses of water.

- If you feel hungry, drink water. Scientists reported that just two 8-ounces glasses of water is an effective weight loss strategy because many times when you feel hungry you are actually thirsty. So, drink water and see if that fills you up before eating anything. You may be pleasantly surprised! This is a link to the article: http://www.acs.org/content/acs/en/pressroom/newsreleases/2010/august/clinical-trial-confirms-effectiveness-of-simple-appetite-control-method.html

- Eliminate soft drinks and fruit juices—they are loaded with sugar. Do not drink diet soda because research indicates that it makes you crave sugar and increases abdominal fat. Here is the link to the article: http://www.medicaldaily.com/4-dangerous-effects-artificial-sweeteners-your-health-247543

- Do not microwave your food or beverages because the microwave alters the food and has been found to decrease hemoglobin and raise bad cholesterol. Read further evidence in this article: http://www.mercola.com/article/microwave/hazards2.htm

- Do not use margarine because it most likely contains trans-fat which increases the risk of heart disease and free radicals which contribute to numerous health problems including cancer and heart disease. Instead use organic butter, olive oil, and coconut oil.

- Do not use artificial sweeteners because people who frequently consume sugar substitutes may be at an increased risk of excessive weight gain, metabolic syndrome, type 2 diabetes, and cardiovascular disease. For further information read this article: http://www.medicaldaily.com/4-dangerous-effects-artificial-sweeteners-your-health-247543

- Substitute sugar with a healthy sweetener like stevia, which is an herb. It should be purchased in a health food store because Truvia and other popular stevia products at the grocery store are too refined. Another option is local honey. However, honey does raise your blood sugar level. I use a powder form of stevia for baking. Also, I have found a natural sweetener that has zero calories and rates zero on the glycemic index. It is Lakanto Monkfruit Sweetener (http://www.lakanto.com/) which is made from monk fruit.

- Curb sweet cravings by adding a teaspoon of raw, unfiltered, unpasteurized apple cider vinegar to a cup of water and a couple of drops of stevia.

- Limit milk products because they are inflammatory and cause mucus formation. If you are lactose intolerant, like me, do not eat milk products. However, if you do, take a Lactaid tablet to help with digestion.

Last year, I taught *The Daniel Plan* http://store.danielplan.com/group-study/?sort=featured&page=1 by Rick Warren, which recommended you stop eating sugar, wheat, and milk products for one week. Then you reintroduce one of those foods at a time to determine any adverse effects. Every time I reintroduced dairy products, I had additional phlegm and post-nasal drip. I realized milk products caused inflammation in my system. It is important for you to figure out what may be causing an inflammatory response in your body. Yoga will help you to become more in tune with your body and how it is functioning.

- Buy organic fruits and vegetables. Some medical literature claims inflammation is the root of chronic disease. Where do you think inflammation comes from? It is from something we put into our bodies and most likely from the food we ingest. There are all sorts of chemicals and additives in our food today. However, a vegetable or piece of fruit does not have those artificial additives except for the pesticides and herbicides that are sprayed on them. That is why I buy organic.

- Be sure you are getting enough fiber. You should have a bowel movement at least once a day. As you increase the fruits and vegetables in your diet, this will not be a problem. However, during this transitional phase, supplement with oxygenated magnesium, ground flaxseed, or other natural fiber supplements from a health food store. During the first three days that you wean yourself off all the white stuff, the Candida in your gut is dying and this 'die off' might make you feel ill like you are getting the flu. Therefore, it is imperative that you do not get constipated during this initial period, so take additional fiber to get the dead Candida out of your body. This will decrease your feeling of illness.

- Replace undesirable ingredients with whole foods. *The Daniel Plan Cookbook* by Rick Warren provides a chart with "Foods and Ingredients to Avoid" and suggested replacements. I will list a few from this book:

  - Replace sugary snacks with nuts, nut butter, dark chocolate, or plain Greek yogurt with berries.

  - Replace condiments and sauces containing MSG or high-fructose corn syrup with spices, vinegar, and herbs.

  - Replace candy with dried fruit.

  - Replace table salt with Kosher or sea salt.

  - Replace fried foods with baked foods.

Here are some of my healthy eating ideas:

- Make homemade granola from oats. For breakfast, I add fresh berries to a bowl of granola.

- Make or buy a flavorful dip like hummus or guacamole to eat with a platter of fresh vegetables. -Substitute beans for meat for some meals.

- Squeeze a slice of lemon and two drops of stevia into a glass of water. It is like having fresh lemonade!

- Boil eggs and keep them in the refrigerator for a snack.

Please try not to be overwhelmed by all of this information. Think of your eating as the 80/20 percent rule. If you eat healthy 80% of the time and not so healthy 20% of the time this will probably be an improvement.

Chapter 16

GUT HEALTH

If you are a carboholic and crave sugar, alcohol, and all that white stuff, then you could have an imbalance in the flora of your gut. If your gut is not healthy, you are not healthy. An excellent resource that will explain what occurs when you have an imbalance is the *Body Ecology Diet* by Donna Gates. Check out her website https://bodyecology.com/.

I had candidiasis (an overgrowth of yeast) I had candidiasis (an overgrowth of yeast) in my gut after having an abscessed tooth, antibiotics, and steroids. Candidiasis is like having a monster growing inside of you, and you don't even know it. It begins to grow roots into the lining of your GI tract and makes you crave carbs because that is what it eats. It is extremely hard to stop this monster's cravings and to kill it, but I did and you can too!

To kill the overgrowth of yeast I stopped eating the following foods for eight months: sugar, fruit, all the white stuff, and I had to limit my alcohol consumption to vodka because it is distilled not fermented. I was successful, but I still cannot eat foods with high sugar content or the candida starts to grow again. I also took large doses of probiotics (up to 100 billion units/day) during that eight months. Today, I still take probiotics but not such a high dosage.

Like I said, I eat to live and to live a healthy, bountiful life. Remember to evaluate every single thing you put into your mouth. Is it alive or is it dead?

Resources

The Daniel Plan: 40 Days to a Healthier Life and *The Daniel Plan Cookbook* by Rick Warren, Daniel Amen MD, Mark Hyman MD

Body Ecology Diet by Donna Gates

Grain Brain by David Perlmutter MD

Wheat Belly by William Davis MD

The Eat Right 4 Your Type by Dr. Peter D'Adamo

If you have cancer, diabetes, or a life threatening disease I recommend trying the Hallelujah Diet at http://www.myhdiet.com/what-is-the-hallelujah-diet/.

Notes

Chapter 1

Mackay, 1928-29, 74-75.

Thomas McEvilley, *Anthropology and Aesthetics*, "An Archaeology of Yoga" (The President and Fellows of Harvard College), 44.

Ulrica Norberg, *Hatha Yoga: The Body's Path to Balance, Focus, and Strength* (New York, New York: Skyhorse Publishing 2008), 17-19.

Chapter 3

Timothy McCall, M.D., *Yoga Journal*, "38 Health Benefits of Yoga" (Cruz Bay Publishing, Inc. 2007), 3-12. http://www.yogajournal.com/article/health/count-yoga-38-ways-yoga-keeps-fit/ June 2016.

Chapter 4

Fernando Pages Ruiz, *Yoga Journal*, "What Science Can Teach Us About Flexibility" (Cruz Bay Publishing, Inc. 2007). http://www.yogajournal.com/article/practice-section/what-science-can-teach-us-about-flexibility/ June 2016.

Kim Innes, PhD, *Journal of Alzheimer's Disease*, "Simple Mind-Body Therapies Shown to Improve Subjective Cognitive Decline, a Pre-Clinical Stage of Alzheimer's Disease" (Amsterdam, IOS Press), June 7, 2016. http://www.j-alz.com/content/simple-mind-body-therapies-shown-improve-subjective-cognitive-decline-pre-clinical-stage June 2016.

Ann Brenoff, *The Huffington Post: Sleep + Wellness,* "Yoga Can Help Improve Memory For Those At Risk For Alzheimer's" (The Huffington Post),May10,2016.http://www.huffingtonpost.com/entry/yoga-reduces-risk-of-alzheimers-says-study_us_5730a855e4b0bc9cb0475be4   June 2016.

Julie T. Lusk, *Yoga Meditations: Timeless Mind-Body Practices for Awakening* (Duluth, Minnesota, Whole Person Associates 2005), 13, 16.

Chapter 14

Dale E. Bredesen Reversal of Cognitive Decline: A Novel Therapeutic Program. Aging. 2014.

Dale E. Bredesen, Edwin C. Amos , Jonathan Canick , Mary Ackerley , Cyrus Raji , Milan Fiala, and Jamila Ahdidan Reversal of cognitive decline in Alzheimer's disease. Aging. June 2016.

William Davis MD, *Wheat Belly* (New York, New York, Rodale Inc.), 8-9.

Brenda Davy, *American Chemical Society (ACS),* "Clinical Trial Confirms effectiveness of Simple Appetite Control Method" August 23 2010. http://www.acs.org/content/acs/en/pressroom/newsreleases/2010/august/clinical-trial-confirms-effectiveness-of-simple-appetite-control-method.html June 2016.

Swithers SE, Patterson NA, *Trends in Endocrinology & Metabolism,* "Artificial sweeteners produce the counterintuitive effect of inducing metabolic derangement" 2013. http://www.medicaldaily.com/4-dangerous-effects-artificial-sweeteners-your-health-247543 May 2016.

Tom Valentine "The Proven Dangers of Microwaves." NEXUS Magazine (April-May '95). Volume 2, #25. http://www.mercola.com/article/microwave/hazards2.htm May 2016.

Yoga Posture Index

✓ 23. Downward Dog

24. Low Lunge

25. Camel

26. Yoga Mudra

27. Cleansing Breath

28. Squat

29. Standing Forward Bend

30. Standing Forward Bend with Leg Clasp and Halfway Lift

31. Mountain

32. Half Moon Side Bend

33. Standing Abdominal Lifts

34. Kegel

✓ 35. Warrior I

✓ 36. Warrior II

37. Standing Side Yoga Mudra

38. Posture Clasp

✓ 39. Triangle

✓ 40. Tree

41. Warrior III

42. Dancer

43. Half Locust

✓ 44. Cobra

✓ 45. Plank

46. Locust

47. Bow

✓ 48. Child's Pose

49. Double Leg Raises

50. Boat

51. Reclining Spinal Twist (Two Knee Variation)

52. Supine Reach Through (Variation)

53. Bridge

54. Shoulder Stand

55. Fish

56. Lying Spinal Twist (One Leg Variation)

57. Alternate Nostril Breath

58. Corpse Pose

59. Single Knee Hug

60. Knee Hug

About the Author

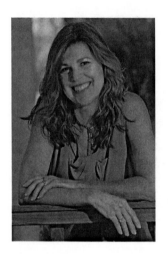

Susan Neal is a certified yoga instructor with over 30 years' experience in practicing and teaching yoga. As a pursuer of ultimate health, Susan merged her practice of yoga with her spiritual practice of Christianity. Founder of Scripture Yoga, Susan recites theme-based Scripture verses during her yoga classes. She published *Scripture Yoga: 21 Bible Lessons for Christian Yoga Classes* and two sets of Scripture Yoga Cards, "How to Receive God's Peace" and "Fruit of the Spirit."

She produced two Christian yoga DVDs, *God's Mighty Angels* and *What the Bible Says About Prayer*. You can purchase these products at http://christianyoga.com.

Since 2004, Susan has taught a free Scripture Yoga class every week at Woodbine United Methodist Church in Pace, Florida. Additionally, she enjoys being a speaker and yoga teacher at women's retreats. If you would like Susan to lead a yoga class at your retreat, please contact her at SusanNeal@Bellsouth.net.

Additionally, Susan produced a hospice CD, *Bedside Encouragement: When You Don't Know How to Say Goodbye,* which was designed to provide peace and comfort to those receiving hospice care. It would make an appropriate gift for someone who recently lost a loved one or has been diagnosed with a terminal illness. You can purchase this CD at HospiceCD.com.

You can follow Susan on:

https://www.instagram.com/scriptureyoga/
https://twitter.com/SusanNealYoga
https://www.pinterest.com/SusanNealYoga/
https://www.facebook.com/ScriptureYoga/
or her YouTube channel at https://www.youtube.com/c/
SusanNealScriptureYoga

I created a Beginner Yoga Class video for you, so you can watch how to perform many of the yoga poses in this book. Enjoy the free Beginner Yoga Class here: http://christianyoga.com/BeginnerYogaVideo

If this book enhanced your yoga practice, would you please take a few minutes to add a book review on Amazon? Simple go to this link: https://www.amazon.com/dp/B01L9UIT70. Book reviews are like gold to authors. Thank you!

CPSIA information can be obtained
at www.ICGtesting.com
Printed in the USA
LVOW10s0920160717

541531LV00006B/355/P